Improving Your Health With Vitamin C

by Ruth Adams
and
Frank Murray

Preventive Health
Library
Series

Larchmont Books
New York

First printing: June, 1978

IMPROVING YOUR HEALTH WITH VITAMIN C

Copyright © Larchmont Books, 1978

ISBN 0-915962-23-3

Printed in the United States of America

LARCHMONT BOOKS
6 East 43rd Street
New York, N.Y. 10017
Tel., 212-949-0800

Contents

CHAPTER 1

Your Need for Vitamin C

IT'S A HORROR STORY to stand your hair on end. And, if somebody on the hospital staff had not finally decided to ask the patient what she usually ate, chances are she would have died on the operating table along about the tenth or eleventh time they opened up her abdomen to find out why she kept bleeding internally.

It started in April 1967, **when this 48-year-old woman came to her doctor complaining of excessive menstrual flow for one year and abdominal pain for the past five weeks.** The doctor asked if she had had any excessive bleeding with a tooth extraction or any complication of childbirth. She hadn't. She didn't show any **black and blue marks which might indicate something wrong with her vitamin C intake.** The only drug she was taking was aspirin for intermittent headaches.

The doctors found her abdomen distended but could find no evidence of the blood-containing tumors called angiomas.

They decided she must have endometriosis (the presence of endometrial tissue in abnormal locations). On April 26, 1967 they operated and found a lot of blood in her abdomen. They didn't know what was causing it, but, just in case, they removed her uterus, her ovaries and her appendix. Her ovaries showed signs of hemorrhaging.

While convalescing the patient suffered from bloating, belching, indigestion and cramping abdominal pain for several months after she was discharged from the hospital. Four months later, she was admitted again with cramping pain and rapidly increasing abdominal distention. The doctors decided she must have a bowel obstruction. So on August 4, 1967, they operated again and found a small twist in her bowel which they straightened out. She had been bleeding internally, however, and they noticed a number of places oozing blood. They cut these out and cauterized them.

In September, 1968, this same patient again complained of cramping pain and abdominal distention. They stuck a diagnostic needle into her abdomen and, sure enough, found blood. They operated once again and there was unclotted blood all about, along with cysts, some filled with blood, others filled with fluid. They "deflated" the cysts and sewed her up again.

In November, 1968, and January, 1969, the patient again suffered from abdominal distention. Another needle produced considerable blood from her abdomen. They gave her a battery of tests trying to determine what could be causing her trouble. No parts of the puzzle seemed to fit into place to form a reliable diagnosis.

So on January 24, 1969, they operated on her again and, sure enough, drew out quite a lot of blood that was just floating around in her abdomen. Her spleen contained some blood tumors. So the surgeons removed her spleen and sewed her up again. Then all the tests were repeated—bone marrow tests and every imaginable test of blood function. All tests were normal. Well, they decided, she must be suffering from hidden cancer in some unsuspected place and it seemed unlikely that they could locate it. They discharged her from the hospital.

In May, 1969, she once again had abdominal distention. Blood tests indicated that she was bleeding internally. This time the doctors decided it must be her pancreas that was acting up. So on May 14 they operated again and found, yes, lots of old blood which was apparently causing her trouble. They removed the pancreas and discharged her from the hospital.

In March, 1971, "the patient was free from disease," says the *Journal of the American Medical Association* (March 28, 1977), reporting on this medical incident. The article goes on to say, **"Questioning prompted the suspicion that her diet was deficient in fresh fruits and vegetables."** No explanation is given for why nobody had ever questioned her about her diet before this. It is apparently taken for granted by these doctors, as by most doctors apparently, that what we eat and do not eat has nothing whatever to do with our health.

So they tested her blood for vitamin C and found that it was all but non-existent. They gave her 1,000 milligrams of vitamin C a day and told her to go on taking that much every day. By 1976, she reported in again and they asked her if she had been taking her vitamin C. Well, no, she hadn't. Sure enough, her blood showed almost no vitamin C once again.

This time they convinced her she must continue taking the vitamin C and the internal bleeding has not happened again. Say the two physicians from a California hospital who made this report in the *JAMA*, "The salutary outcome (of this case) can be interpreted in terms of the vascular effects of vitamin C. Deficiency leads to formation of defective ground substance in collagen, the support material of vascular structures. Serious deficiency leads to vascular disruption and bleeding. Moreover, if superimposed on vasculature already flawed, bleeding eventuates more readily. This process, however, is reversible. . . . **Subclinical scurvy**

7

should be considered whenever bleeding develops in angiomatous (blood-tumor-forming) patients."

It seems to us that the above incident gives a very good indication why medical and health care costs are increasing astronomically. It's impossible even to estimate the cost of this one patient's medical and surgical bills—$50,000? $100,000? Half a million? **The entire cost in agony and in dollars, to say nothing of the crippling of this woman through loss of body organs, could have been prevented by the use of a few dollars worth of vitamin C per month.** That's all that was necessary. Who knows how many people who come to hospitals or doctors' offices might be cured easily and painlessly with the same few dollars worth of a harmless substance?

Is there any indication that any physician will take to heart the recommendations of the California doctors that this usually fatal kind of internal bleeding be treated first with vitamin C, or at least that the patient's vitamin C status be determined before heroic measures are undertaken, since there is apparently no way to know who is suffering from scurvy without testing blood for vitamin C content? What's your guess?

Many other questions come to our mind in regard to this patient. Does she smoke? How many aspirins did she consume trying to get rid of her headaches? Aspirin is a well-known destroyer of vitamin C. In sunny California, where oranges grow on the trees free for the picking in almost every backyard, and gardens and truck farms fill every warm corner, how did it happen that this woman just never ate any fruits or vegetables, which are the only dependable sources of vitamin C in foods? How much more likely it seems that in colder parts of the country and in localities which are economically stressed, such vitamin deficiency is common and such misdiagnoses result in much unnecessary surgery and drug therapy?

The above story becomes even more depressing in the light of three other articles we uncovered recently discussing

8

malnutrition in relation to hospital patients. *The Lancet* for March 26, 1977 reported on **the nutritional status of 105 surgical patients. The doctors found gross nutritional deficiencies in the group as a whole and especially among patients who were still in the hospital more than a week after major surgery.** Why does this surprise the doctors? Have they never heard that stresses use up nutritional elements very rapidly and that, the more stress, the more nutritional support should be given?

Geriatrics for February, 1977 reported on the "poorly understood surgical risk factor in aged cardiac patients." **Patients being prepared for surgery should be given supernutritious diets,** say the authors, both intravenously and orally.

And the *Journal of the American Medical Association* for March 28, 1977 reported that growing concern over patient nutrition was evident at a recent medical meeting "where a panel of experts examined the fruit-juice-jello-missed-meals syndrome." **"There is no pathological process or therapy in which you can expect a patient to do better when he's malnourished than when he is well nourished,"** said a Texas physician. A masterpiece of understatement, we would call this.

He went on to say, "Weigh your patients. **X-ray therapy is one of the most severe catabolic stresses to a patient that we've seen.** Someone has to watch these patients to make sure they can withstand the combined insults of the disease and the therapy." Lack of energy in a patient is a signal to "stop; do not proceed" until the patient is feeling energetic and well nourished. Other physicians commented on the **frequency of protein malnutrition**—certain amino acids being missing, which may lead to bed sores, poor wound healing, decreased resistance to infection and many other unacceptable sequels of surgery.

"If you operate on the bowel of a malnourished patient, it falls apart," said a Cornell surgeon. "If you operate on the heart of a malnourished patient, it falls apart." Other panel members warned against impatience in nutritional rehabilitation. It is a long haul. One physician pointed out that it may take months to return to good nutritional health a patient who has lost 15 to 20 grams of nitrogen daily while in the hospital.

"**The clear message to physicians is that no patient should be hospitalized without an adequate nutrition profile,**" said a Harvard professor. "Don't eat for the rest of the day, and see how well *you* feel."

Two African scientists reported in *Nature* for August 4, 1972 that **vitamin C is low in the blood corpuscles of women who take oral contraceptives.** The lack of vitamin C appeared to be related to the fact that the vitamin C was taken by mouth, for, when the hormone was injected, the levels of vitamin C were not affected. Women who take The Pill should get all the protection they can by increasing their intake of various vitamins, including several B vitamins and vitamin C.

Dr. T. S. Wilson at Barncoose Hospital in Redruth, England, surveyed the vitamin C status of elderly patients being admitted to his hospital. Then he noted what course their health took from then on. He reported in *Gerontologia Clinica*, Vol. 14, page 17, 1972, that **the elderly men and women with higher levels of vitamin C upon admission had longer lives than those with lower levels of vitamin C.** The low vitamin C levels did not seem to produce any specific illness or condition of ill health. But, just the same, the patients with lower levels of the vitamin died sooner from all diseases.

It has been speculated that vitamin C might function to control fertility. Could we possibly use this eminently safe vitamin as a birth control pill? asked Dr. M. H. Briggs. His suggestion appeared in *The Lancet*, the British medical journal. In a later issue (November 17, 1973), Dr. Abram Hoffer of Canada answered him with a resounding "No." Said Dr. Hoffer, "I have been giving large doses of vitamin C (2 to 10 grams per day) for over 20 years, and have not been aware of any lowering of fertility among my patients (over 3,000). A 10-minute search of my files produced the following women patients, who all became pregnant while taking ascorbic acid."

Dr. Hoffer then describes the cases of four women taking from two to three grams of vitamin C daily. All of them became pregnant during this treatment.

"In 20 years of experience," says Dr. Hoffer, "I have not seen any of the following: post-ascorbic acid scurvy, withdrawal symptoms, increase in incidence of collagen diseases or oxalate urinary stones. My experience on over 3,000 cases provides no support for the hypothesis."

Dr. Hoffer is talking about various theories that have been advanced **on massive doses of vitamin C**. Some scientists have theorized that people who take large doses of vitamin C may have symptoms of scurvy when they stop taking such large doses. Other scientists have talked about the possibility of withdrawal symptoms—that is, some kind of unpleasant symptoms such as drug addicts suffer when they stop taking their drugs. Or, according to some theorists, large doses of vitamin C might possibly bring on some such diseases as arthritis or perhaps kidney or bladder stones. **Never, in all his 3,000 patients taking from 2,000 to 3,000 milligrams of vitamin C daily has Dr. Hoffer ever found any such complaints.**

Dr. Hoffer is one of the first physicians on this continent to use massive doses of vitamin C, as well as several of the B vitamins, in treating his patients suffering from **schizophrenia**, the mental disorder which has many of the same symptoms as pellagra, the disease of vitamin B deficiency.

A British physician has, for a number of years, been using vitamin C in the treatment of patients at a mental hospital. Dr. G. Milner's interest was roused when he read research indicating that **anxiety and excitement tend to destroy the body's supply of vitamin C.** He found, too, that mental patients suffering from schizophrenia have lower levels of vitamin C in their blood than normal people, even though

11

they are getting the same amount in their food.

He knows, too, that there is a condition called "**sub-scurvy," in which individuals feel tired, depressed, irritable and complain of vague ill-health**. They do not have a full-blown case of scurvy with hemorrhaging and painful muscles and all the other symptoms of this devastating disease. But one would certainly not say they are in good health.

Why not, said Dr. Milner, try to clarify the situation in regard to vitamin C and mental health, to discover whether lack of this nutrient may have something to do with some of the complaints of mentally ill patients—tiredness, depression, etc? So he set up an experiment in a mental hospital, with the cooperation of 40 male patients, some of whom had been in the hospital for as long as 45 years.

Studying these men before the experiment began, he found that 12 of them already had symptoms of vitamin C deficiency, which no one had apparently thought of any importance. They had indigestion, tiny hemorrhages on the scalp, bleeding gums and rather horny skin. **Those patients who were given vitamin C during the test improved, while they were taking the vitamin. All the symptoms disappeared.**

The doctor divided the patients into two groups, each of whom took a measured dose of a liquid every day for three weeks. Twenty of them were taking one gram of vitamin C; the others were taking nothing but flavored water. No one, including the doctors, patients and nurses, knew which patients had been taking the vitamin until the test was completed. Throughout the test, all patients were given psychiatric tests which indicate the patient's frame of mind—whether he is still depressed, manic, paranoid, and so forth. Throughout these three weeks, too, nurses and other doctors made notes on their impressions of each patient's condition—whether or not he had improved.

After the test was completed, **it was found that the patients taking vitamin C had improved considerably,** both in the tests and in the opinion of those caring for them. Even more important, said Dr. Milner, is his discovery that **these patients were short on vitamin C, although they were eating a well-planned diet in which there was apparently enough vitamin C for a well person.**

These people simply had a greater need for vitamin C than the rest of us. Did their state of "subscurvy" contribute to their mental condition? We do not know. But we do know that they improved immeasurably within three weeks when they were given a daily massive dose of vitamin C, so that all their body tissues were saturated with the vitamin.

We found in the medical literature a report on a New Zealand doctor who has been conducting similar experiments. He, too, has found that **mentally ill patients need much more vitamin C than well people.** As their mental condition becomes worse, and excitement and anxiety mount, they need even more vitamin C.

Dr. Wilson Dalton of Shelbyville, Indiana uses massive doses of vitamin C to treat **viral diseases.** In an article in the *Journal of the Indiana State Medical Association,* he tells of patients with viral pneumonia, bronchitis, sinusitis, flu, hepatitis—**all of whom responded almost miraculously to massive doses of a preparation of vitamin C, along with the B vitamins,** which this doctor injected daily.

Dr. E. Cheraskin and his group of researchers at the University of Alabama have developed a unique method of investigating important nutritional matters. They deal with a large group of professional people—dentists and their wives—who have agreed to give information and answer questionnaires about their eating habits and other aspects of life. When the replies from 400 or so such individuals come in, they are fed into a computer and highly significant answers come to light.

In an article in the *Journal of the American Geriatrics Society* for March, 1976, Dr. Cheraskin and his colleagues take up the possible relationship of **fatigue and lack of enough vitamin C.** They turned up some fascinating facts.

13

First they searched the scientific literature on the subject and found very little that was helpful. It has been known for years that when volunteers are deliberately made deficient in vitamin C to the point where they develop scurvy, a progressive feeling of fatigue develops by the beginning of the third month. These are people who are getting enough of all other nutrients. Just vitamin C is lacking.

Other researchers have found that manual workers can work at apparent top efficiency when they are deprived of vitamin C for as long as eight weeks. Giving them 75 milligrams of the vitamin daily did nothing to improve their performance.

In a study of air force personnel in 1970, physicians found that a daily supplement of 1,000 milligrams of vitamin C apparently had no effect on the endurance of these men while they were performing in various sports. The doctors admitted that results might have been different had the men been older or if they had been tested on something other than contact sports. These doctors suggested that double-blind tests be done to get a better answer.

Dr. Cheraskin and his colleagues decided to seek an answer from the professional group with which they have worked for many years. **They sent questionnaires to 411 dentists and their wives.** They asked them to list everything they ate in a given period of time, including the vitamin supplements they take.

Then they sent them something called the Cornell Medical Index Health Questionnaire, which has been in use for some time as a reliable measure of many aspects of health—good and bad. The questions asked of these 411 people were aimed to discover how tired they are daily and how much they complain of fatigue. No other questions were asked. The Alabama scientists did not inquire into anything else these people eat or don't eat, nor did they ask how much sleep or rest they got, how fatiguing their daily work is or anything else pertaining to their diet and way of life. Just how much vitamin C they get daily (calculated from food, drink and supplements) and how tired they get.

Eighty-one of the people questioned consume less than 100 milligrams of vitamin C daily. Three hundred thirty people get more than 400 milligrams of vitamin C daily. The second group reported just about half the amount of fatigue the first group reported.

Now, of course, it's perfectly possible that those people among the 411 who get the most vitamin C are also the people who guard their health more carefully in other ways as well. Maybe they plan better diets. Maybe they eat more protein with less sugar and refined starches. Maybe they also take other vitamin supplements as well as mineral supplements and this influences their replies. Maybe they also get more exercise, more sleep and rest. We do not know.

The only nutritional element investigated was the amount of vitamin C they get every day. The only other health characteristic investigated was how tired they are. The two seemed to correlate without a shadow of a doubt. **The people who got the most vitamin C complained of the least fatigue.** Dr. Cheraskin and his colleagues say they believe this test might prove helpful in detecting ill health at an early stage. Presumably people who tire easily are more likely to be ill.

It seems to us that this test is a good indication of further help we may be able to get from vitamin C—more stamina, less fatigue; more endurance, more ability to stand up to every day's crises and problems. There's no reason not to try it.

Dr. Cheraskin's book, *Psychodietetics*, is a fascinating book on the subject of nutrition and mental and emotional health. It is crammed with tests you can give yourself to discover just how good your own mental condition is and how good your own nutritional health is.

Dr. Cheraskin and his co-author, Dr. W. M. Ringsdorf, Jr., give recommendations for achieving some of the following by good nutrition and nutritional supplements: relieving nervousness and irritability, alleviating some of the

15

symptoms of senility and old age, including loss of memory, avoiding loss of nutrients from unwise dieting and taking drugs (both prescription and over-the-counter drugs) and finally how to achieve the optimal diet, in terms of daily meals and supplements.

A recommended battery of vitamins and minerals in terms of the optimal amount to be taken every day is surely one of the most helpful aids we can have. These two experts in the field outline just such a diet and supplement program, telling you what to avoid and what to seek out. The paperback edition of *Psychodietetics* is published by Bantam Books, 666 Fifth Avenue, New York City. It costs $1.95.

Vitamin C for hangovers? Well, that's the word from scientists at Jefferson Medical College and the Veterans Hospital in Coatesville, Pa. They have found that vitamin C and vitamin B1 (thiamine) given to laboratory rats, along with the amino acid cysteine, which is found in all high-protein foods, give good protection against harm from large amounts of alcohol. Acetaldehyde, a poisonous chemical 10 to 30 times more toxic than alcohol, is formed when liquor breaks down in the body. It is also a toxic component of cigarette smoke. It is associated with aging. It can cause death by damaging the liver, kidneys, heart, brain and other organs. So the combination of a drink and a cigarette appears to be much more harmful than either of them alone.

Experiments begun in 1974 by Dr. Herbert Sprince and his colleagues at the college show that vitamin C, thiamine and cysteine neutralize or reduce the damage done by acetaldehyde. Some animals which were near death from these toxic effects recovered. Said Dr. Sprince, "Our findings demonstrate for the first time that direct protective action against acetaldehyde toxicity and lethality can be obtained with certain naturally occurring metabolites, namely ascorbic acid, cysteine and thiamine preferably in combination at reduced dose levels."

They added the precaution that further research in animals is necessary before the long-term use of these

16

compounds in high doses for human beings can be considered. Vitamin C is harmless in massive doses, as we know. Thiamine is a B vitamin, also soluble in water, hence excreted harmlessly if too much is taken. As is the case with all B vitamins, however, it would be best to accompany any large doses of individual B vitamins with members of the entire B complex.

Cysteine is not one of the "essential" amino acids—that is, the ones which we must get in food since we cannot manufacture them ourselves. The healthy body manufactures some cysteine. But larger supplies are available from all high protein foods: meat, poultry, eggs, dairy products and seed foods chiefly. So take your thiamine and vitamin C with a slab of cheese on real wholegrain bread. And we would also recommend doing your very best to stop drinking and smoking.

A recent study in Italy has shown that, **in guinea pigs at least, the one organ of the body which is most affected by lack of vitamin C is the brain.** In *Orthomolecular Psychiatry*, Dr. Linus Pauling and other specialists presented their theory that a kind of scurvy of the brain might be a leading cause of schizophrenia, our most prevalent mental illness. Scurvy is the disease resulting from lack of vitamin C.

Four scientists at the University of Padova in Italy reported in the *International Journal of Vitamin and Nutrition Research* that they had withheld vitamin C from guinea pigs until the animals developed a chronic condition of vitamin C deficiency—a sort of subclinical scurvy. Then they measured the amounts of various essential substances in their brains.

They found, sure enough, that there were very definite and important changes which would be bound to affect many brain and nerve functions in the lives of these animals. If the same is true of human beings—and there seems no reason why it should not be—plain lack of enough vitamin C might certainly be a partial cause of many mental disorders, both serious and minor, both acute and chronic.

17

The liver of guinea pigs—like the liver of human beings—stores vitamin C. But throughout the Italian experiments it was found that changes in the brain were more important than changes in the liver. From this the scientists conclude that the brain is that part of living creatures which suffers most from lack of vitamin C. They pointed out one fact which surfaces in many studies of mental disorder. The copper content of the brain is increased when vitamin C is lacking. "It is well known," say these scientists, "that neurologic and psychiatric damage usually follows increase in brain copper concentrations."

Guinea pigs need so much vitamin C for good health that an equivalent amount for the much heavier adult human being would be 5 to 15 grams a day—that is, 5,000 to 15,000 milligrams. And the officially recommended amount for good health is a measly 45 milligrams! Since 1949 biologists have known that the wild gorilla, eating fresh tropical foods all day, gets as much as 4,000 to 5,000 milligrams of vitamin C a day. This suggests, says Dr. Pauling in *Executive Health* (Vol. IX, No. 5), **"That one or two grams (1,000 to 2,000 milligrams) might be needed by man for the best health."**

In his article, Dr. Pauling goes on to talk about **the possibility of vitamin C being powerful against other viruses than the ones which produce the common cold.** He reminds us that we have almost no drugs that conquer viruses. He thinks that taking one or two grams of vitamin C a day might decrease one's chances of getting some viral disease. Still more protection might be provided, he says, by increasing the amount you take during times of exposure.

Dr. Pauling agrees with all those scientists who have worked with vitamin C that answers to these terribly important questions can come only if our government breaks down its prejudice against this kind of research and gives some financial grants to the scientists who are eager to work on vitamin C. Scientific work must be supported by financial grants. The scientific and health branches of our federal government are simply not interested.

The *Washington Post* reported on December 22, 1975 that

Dr. Pauling is unable to get federal funds for work on treating cancer with vitamin C. He works closely with a Scots researcher, Ewan Cameron, as we learn in another chapter, whose work with cancer patients and vitamin C has been published in scientific journals around the world.

A Rutgers University researcher was refused federal funds for work aimed at reducing hardening of the arteries with vitamin C. He had shown, working with rabbits, great reduction in the plaques which shut off blood flow in the arteries, when vitamin C was given. Now he cannot continue his work. The Washington bureaucrats are more interested in developing new drugs.

Dr. Jorgen Schlegel of Tulane Medical School has used vitamin C in fighting bladder cancer. Dr. Eli Seifter was the first to demonstrate that vitamin A could be used against tumors of viral origin. Both these distinguished men have been refused federal funds to continue their work. The National Cancer Institute has $800 million of taxpayers' money to pursue research. Less than six million of it went for nutritional research in 1975.

In *Executive Health* for December, 1975, Dr. Pauling tells us of a study in San Mateo County, California, which showed that **people with a low intake of vitamin C had a death rate from all causes—mainly heart disease and cancer—which was 2 1/2 times that of people who took some vitamin C.** The study involved 577 people—all over the age of 50. And the protective power of vitamin C showed itself, even though the amount of vitamin C taken was only about 100 milligrams a day!

Says Dr. Pauling, **"I am now willing to predict that people who take the optimum amount of vitamin C may well have, at each age, only one-quarter as much illness and chance of dying as those who do not take extra vitamin C.** This way of improving one's health will not, I believe, be ignored much longer."

CHAPTER 2

How Much Vitamin C Do You Need?

IN THE YEARS since massive doses of vitamin C have been prescribed by many physicians and psychiatrists, those researchers who dislike the idea that just plain vitamins can treat or prevent illness have been telling us that we're all wasting our money. Their belittling, disparaging comments suggest that all vitamin C over a dose of perhaps 30 to 100 milligrams is excreted almost immediately in the urine. So all we "faddists" are doing, say these detractors, is to create very expensive urine for ourselves.

At the same time they tell us that vitamin C may bring us harm. They never explain just how this perfectly natural substance, which plays many important roles in the human body, could harm us if it is indeed all excreted within a few hours. Harmful things are usually substances that are stored in the body, accumulating until the total amount overwhelms us.

Those researchers who regularly use vitamin C in very large amounts continually search for some evidence of harm from the vitamin and have been unable to find any. The detractors, too, have never been able to produce any verified cases where large doses of vitamin C have brought anything but benefit.

Now we have a very significant record of tests done in a school for mentally disturbed patients who were getting extremely large amounts of vitamin C. Four physicians from the Virginia school write in *The Journal of Orthomolecular Psychiatry*, Volume 5, No. 1, about their very careful tests to determine exactly how much vitamin C is excreted in the urine.

Ninety-one patients getting from 4 to 48 grams of vitamin C daily were tested. This is 4,000 to 48,000 milligrams. Thirty-one of these patients were excreting vitamin C. Sixty of them were not. This means, we must assume, that these 60 people needed that much vitamin C daily, or perhaps needed even more than this, since the vitamin was doing its job in their cells and was consumed in the process.

Four months later these same patients were tested again. Of 99 tests, 20 patients were excreting vitamin C. The rest were not. Apparently the 79 patients needed this much or more vitamin C. Later tests turned up the fact that about one-fourth of the patients were excreting vitamin C. Still later tests revealed that 37 per cent, 25 per cent, 34 per cent, and so on were excreting vitamin C, hence getting more than they apparently needed.

During a later period, 149 new patients were admitted to the school. **Urine tests showed not a particle of vitamin C in the urine of any of these patients. Doesn't this demonstrate clearly that these patients were not getting anywhere near the amount of the vitamin that they needed?** Could this not be, as orthomolecular psychiatrists believe, one of the causes of their mental and emotional illness-lack of enough vitamin C to make up for the very great stress of their illness?

While these tests were going on, the investigators also tested school personnel—the nurses, doctors and administrative officials. Of 25 samples of urine taken, 19 showed ascorbic acid. Six did not. So at least six of these supposedly perfectly well individuals were not getting enough vitamin C

21

to be able to spare any to excrete in their urine.

And what about the potential danger of large doses of vitamin C? In this situation, all patients were being observed constantly. Tests were constantly being given and symptoms were constantly being checked. **Of the entire population of patients who were getting an average of nine grams (9,000 milligrams) of vitamin C daily, not a**

Foods Highest in Vitamin C

Food	Milligrams of Vitamin C
Acerola cherries	1000 milligrams in 100 grams
Asparagus, fresh green	20 in 8 stalks
Beans, green lima	9 in ½ cup
Beet greens, cooked	25 in ½ cup
Broccoli, leaf	90 in ¾ cup
Brussels sprouts	87 in ¾ cup
Cabbage, Chinese, raw	50 in 1 cup
Cabbage, green, raw	50 in 1 cup
Cabbage, inside leaves, raw	50 in 1 cup
Cantaloupe	50 in ½ sm. cantaloupe
Chard, Swiss, cooked	16 in ½ cup
Collards, cooked	70 in ½ cup
Currants, red	40 in 1 cup
Dandelion greens, cooked	18 in 1 cup
Grapefruit, fresh	45 in ½ cup grapefruit
Grapefruit juice, fresh	108 in 1 cup
Grapefruit juice, canned	72 in 1 cup
Guavas	125 in 1 guava
Honeydew melon	90 in ¼ med. honeydew
Kale, cooked	96 in ¾ cup
Kohlrabi	50 in ½ cup
Leeks	25 in ½ cup
Lemon juice	25 in 1 tablespoon
Lime juice	18 in ¼ cup
Liver, beef	30 in 1 slice
Liver, calves	25 in 1 slice
Liver, chicken	25 in ½ cup
Liver, lamb	20 in 1 slice

single symptom of any kind of ill effect could be found.
(The average figure of nine grams means, of course, that many of the patients were getting much higher doses; some were getting lower doses).

Many of the hospital personnel had undoubtedly observed the beneficial results on health from massive doses of vitamin C. Eighteen staff members have been taking from 6

Food	Milligrams of Vitamin C
Loganberries	35 in 1 cup
Mustard greens, cooked	40 in ½ cup
Orange	50 in 1 med. orange
Orange juice, fresh	120 in 1 cup
Orange juice, canned	80 in 1 cup
Parsley	70 in ½ cup
Parsnips	20 in ½ cup
Peas, fresh cooked	40 in 1 cup
Peppers, green	125 in 1 med. pepper
Peppers, pimiento	95 in 2 med. peppers
Persimmon, Japanese	40 in 1 large persimmon
Pineapple, fresh	17 in ⅔ cup
Pineapple juice, canned	25 in 1 cup
Potatoes, sweet	25 in 1 med. potato
Potatoes, white, baked	20 in 1 med. potato
Radishes	25 in 15 large radishes
Raspberries, black	36 in 1 cup
Raspberries, red	50 in 1 cup
Rose hips	500 to 6000 in 100 grams
Rutabagas	26 in ¾ cup
Spinach, cooked	30 in ½ cup
Strawberries, fresh	50 in ½ cup
Tangerines	48 in 2 med. tangerines
Tomatoes, canned	20 in ½ cup
Tomatoes, fresh	25 in 1 med. tomato
Tomato juice, canned	48 in 1 cup
Turnips, cooked	22 in ½ cup
Turnips, raw	30 in 1 med. turnip
Turnip tops, cooked	40 in ½ cup
Watercress	54 in 1 average bunch

to 18 grams of vitamin C daily for periods up to eight years. These are trained personnel: nurses, doctors and so on. **None of them has noticed any unpleasant side effects, any disease or dysfunction since they began taking the vitamin C, hence attributable to these large doses of the vitamin.**

Say the authors, **"The psychiatric patient is under high stress and obviously requires very large doses of ascorbic acid (vitamin C).** The long-term supplementation of ascorbic acid is apparently a very low risk regimen."

Dr. Linus Pauling shattered the complacency of the world of biochemists by proclaiming in his book, *Vitamin C and the Common Cold,* **that most of us may need lots more vitamin C than we are getting**—far, far more than the official recommended daily allowance.

Some learned nutrition experts rushed into print to deny that such could be the case. Why, they said, the official standard for a daily intake of vitamin C is 60 milligrams (it has since been lowered to 45) for a healthy, adult male and you don't see many cases of scurvy around, do you? Scurvy is the classic disease of vitamin C deficiency.

What these critics overlook is that you *do* see many cases of the common cold these days. During the season, very few of us manage to escape some of the symptoms of this rather mysterious ailment, and most of us have three or four colds a year regularly. **Dr. Pauling theorizes in his book that getting as much vitamin C as our inherited need dictates could prevent cold symptoms and, if we succumb to a cold, could prevent the development of complications, as well as shortening the duration of the cold.**

Our individual needs for vitamin C have been the subject of careful investigation by many other scientists. Working with animals, these men have shown that, even in laboratory animals which are bred to be as much alike as possible, individual requirements for vitamins may vary greatly.

"For decades we have known that the lack of vitamin

C causes impairment in many ways: loss of weight, anemia, extreme weakness in muscles including the heart, bones becoming thin and fragile, loosened teeth, and a tendency to hemorrhage into various tissues; in fact, the effects of deficiency are so diverse that practically every organ in the body is affected," says a University of Texas scientist, writing to the editor of *Science*, the official publication of the American Association for the Advancement of Science.

He goes on to say that over the years there have been reports of the benefits of relatively large doses of vitamin C in a wide variety of disorders. One recent report states that **relatively large doses—up to 500 or 1,000 milligrams daily—are effective in treating back difficulties involving the discs and ligaments.**

The scientist, Dr. Roger J. Williams, and his associate, Gary Deason, ask whether some individuals inherently require much larger amounts of vitamin C than the amounts recommended. To help answer this question, they tested more than 100 guinea pigs. Guinea pigs are one animal which, along with human beings, supposedly cannot manufacture their own vitamin C, as most other animals do. They must obtain it in their food.

They gave their guinea pigs eight different dosages of vitamin C and discovered that "individual guinea pigs have highly variable needs" for vitamin C. In other words, some needed far more than others to remain healthy.

"There is every reason to think that this variability carries over to the human species," they said. "Some guinea pigs have the ability to produce their own vitamin C," the authors go on to say, so that they do not need so much in food. Perhaps the same is true of human beings.

"It is our considered opinion," they add, "that, because of lack of attention to individual needs, medical scientists are missing the important practical benefit from the use of vitamins and other nutrients in the treatment of a variety of diseases. In our country, there are very few centers where

25

such possibilities are being explored," Dr. Williams and Deason say.

We agree. And we applaud Dr. Williams' courage and foresight in writing this letter. It is not easy to take up the cudgels for unpopular causes. A professional man takes chances with his future career every time he does so. Vitamins are not being used as Dr. Williams suggests, mostly, we are told, because the drug companies cannot patent them and make huge sums out of selling them under brand names, as they do with drugs.

Another reason, undoubtedly, is that the Food and Drug Administration insists upon proclaiming that all Americans are getting enough of all the vitamins and minerals, if they eat a "well-rounded diet." This is obviously absurd if individual needs are as various as Dr. Williams believes them to be, and has found in his work that they are. At least we who know the facts can use them to create better health for ourselves and our families.

How much vitamin C do you need? That is hard to speculate because we are all different. But the Recommended Daily Dietary Allowances, as issued in 1974 by the Food and Nutrition Board of the National Academy of Sciences-National Research Council are as follows:

Infants (Up to 1 year):	35 milligrams
Children (1 to 10):	40 milligrams
Males (11 and over):	45 milligrams
Females (11 and over):	45 milligrams
Pregnant females:	60 milligrams
Lactating females:	80 milligrams

Where do you get vitamin C besides in food supplements? The accompanying charts show the major sources of this vitamin. Make sure that you include plenty of these vitamin C-rich foods in your meals each day.

CHAPTER 3

Does a Vitamin C Deficiency Cause Cancer?

In June, 1976, Dr. Linus Pauling appeared on the radio in England and made an astounding announcement. **He said that cancer may be a disease of vitamin C deficiency.** He backed up his claim by referring to the work of a Scots physician, which seems to show that **large doses of vitamin C increase the average survival times of terminal cancer patients four-fold**. And, says Dr. Pauling, "vitamin C can sometimes produce quite dramatic remissions in advanced human cancer."

Dr. Pauling says that the first barrier to the malignant growth of a cancer is the ground substance between cells. Vitamin C is essential for maintaining the structural integrity of this material, hence the vitamin must be one of the body's best weapons for fighting cancer. Dr. Pauling believes that the best treatment for cancer is a judicious combination of medical methods that will eradicate the cancer mass: radiation therapy, surgery, chemotherapy, immunotherapy, plus "supportive measures prescribed in the short term to correct biochemical deficiencies, and in the long term to enhance natural resistance to any residual disease."

Cancer patients are known to be seriously depleted of vitamin C, said Dr. Pauling. Short-term treatment should include vitamin C to correct this deficiency just as it includes **supplemental iron to correct accompanying anemia**. In the long-term view, said Dr. Pauling, vitamin C provides "a simple, safe, practical method of enhancing host resistance to malignant disease."

One of the tests on which Dr. Pauling based his theory is the one conducted in a Scottish hospital by a surgeon, Dr. Ewan Cameron, who gave 10 grams of vitamin C daily—that's 10,000 milligrams—to terminal cancer patients who were "untreatable by any conventional method of therapy at the time of entry into supplemental ascorbate (vitamin C) as their only definitive form of medication." In other words, everything that could be done for these patients by orthodox medicine had already been done. Vitamin C was the only medication given them in their last weeks.

Dr. Pauling reported that there were many instances of relief of symptoms—reduced pain which permitted their doctor to discontinue sedatives. Their appetites returned. They had a renewed sense of well being. It seems that doctors are not especially interested in medicines that just make the patient feel better and many doctors apparently believe that vitamin C does indeed increase the general feeling of well being in many ill people. So, they asked, if that's all the vitamin does—what else is new?

What's new, said Dr. Pauling, is that **results of the experiment seemed to indicate that these patients lived significantly longer than normal clinical expectations**, considering how gravely ill they were. The Scots surgeon then got out records of 1,000 other cancer patients in the same hospital and compared them with the records of the 100 patients to whom he had given vitamin C. He carefully matched each of his patients with 10 of those whose records were in hospital files. Matched patients must be the same age, same kind of tumor, same sex and, in the case of the 1,000

28

past patients, must have had no vitamin C treatment.

The results of this comparison showed clearly that **the patients who got the vitamin C lived on the average four times longer than the original 10 patients to whom they were compared.** Of the 100 patients treated with vitamin C, 15 survived longer than a year, compared to only four of the controls. Six terminal patients treated with vitamin C lived more than two years, compared to only two of the controls. Three of those treated with vitamin C lived for three years. None of those not so treated lived longer than 2½ years.

Of the five who survived more than one year, five are still alive including two who have lived for more than four years. Said the surgeon, "they should have died long ago." He said, too, that **8 to 10 per cent of patients who were "clearly dying of cancer and as a result of receiving nothing but ascorbic acid (vitamin C) show quite definite evidence of tumor regression and recovery.** This is infinitely better than spontaneous regression. I have only seen three spontaneous regressions in my working lifetime."

Critics of this study say that next to nothing can be told by case histories from the files of a hospital. One doctor does not mean the same thing another doctor means when he says "untreatable cancer." And maybe these test patients were just getting better care than those 1,000 past patients to whom they were compared. The surgeon admitted that his assistant had visited the patients once every two weeks to be sure they were taking their vitamin C. He admits that this is therapeutic, but, he says, "I don't think she could have made the tumors regress."

One of the critics, Dr. Kurt Hellman of the Imperial Cancer Research Fund in London, admitted that vitamin C probably could be helpful in cancer treatment. He himself has authored a book on cancer which speculated on the possibilities of vitamin C in cancer treatment. He admits that **vitamin C "is supportive and not toxic."** Many cancer patients are old and poorly nourished, he said, so giving them vitamin C could be valuable for that reason alone. So he thinks the idea could "be valuable."

The Scots surgeon says it is difficult to arrange comparisons of this kind on patients in a general hospital. So he may not be able to pursue his ideas further. Then, too, he said, "other researchers have been so conditioned by the thought that we have enough vitamin C in our diet that the surgeon might have trouble selling the idea to other researchers." **Everyone involved admits that the vitamin C treatment is harmless.**

The British publication (*New Scientist*, July 1, 1976) commenting on Dr. Pauling's statements, mentioned a conference at the New York Academy of Science last year at which the conference in general recommended a daily intake of 500 milligrams of vitamin C.

Once you get into a discussion of this highly controversial vitamin, lots of dissenting opinions come to the surface. Some experts feel that large doses of vitamin C might cause kidney stones, although, as we have discussed in another chapter, there is no single such case recorded. And there is **plenty of evidence that vitamin C may prevent kidney and bladder stones, as well as other serious bladder conditions, including cancer.**

Once you get into the question of preventing colds, one scientist who has apparently never tried the vitamin himself announced recently that up to 1,000 milligrams of vitamin C daily will prevent colds, but more than that, he says, decreases the effectiveness of the vitamin. And the same may be true of cancer, says this researcher, Professor Cedric Wilson. Vitamin C must certainly be involved in the body's attempt to "build a wall" around the cancer to prevent it from spreading to other parts of the body. But, he says, by the same token cancer tissue contains more vitamin C than healthy body tissue surrounding it. Therefore, he believes the tumor is bagging most of the vitamin C for its own growth and not leaving enough for the healthy tissues to maintain themselves. He seems to think that giving more vitamin C will just cause the tumor to grow more. It seems evident that patients of the Scots surgeon did not have that experience.

It is interesting that **Dr. Wilson also believes that colds, allergies, rheumatic arthritis, cancer and other diseases decrease the amount of vitamin C available in the body,** so, therefore, we should take large doses of the vitamin "to restore tissue health." Just what the health food movement has been saying all along!

Dr. Pauling believes that the material between cells must be kept healthy in order to prevent cancer. These cells are normally restrained from proliferating and running wild by a complex mechanism involving a substance called physiological hyaluronidase (PHI). **Vitamin C is necessary for the production of this substance.** It is destroyed in the process of building PHI. Given an adequate quantity of vitamin C, says Dr. Pauling, the body could presumably manufacture enough of this important substance to prevent cancer.

The effect of such a treatment would be to "disarm" the cancer cells. They would remain there, but further growth would stop. Perhaps ulcers would heal, pain, hemorrhaging, weakness, emaciation, malnutrition and all other distressing symptoms might be controlled. This explanation derives from what happens in scurvy, the disease of vitamin C deficiency. The substance between the cells breaks down, leading to tissue disruption, ulceration and hemorrhage— "identical to the local changes that occur in the immediate vicinity of neoplastic (cancerous) cells," says Dr. Pauling.

Why should we, the general public, permit any more guessing, discussion, haggling or arguing about this important life and death matter? Everyone involved in this cancer debate agrees that vitamin C in large doses cannot do any harm. For goodness sake, why not use it then, no matter what else is being done—first to prevent cancer, and as part of the treatment of cancer—any cancer, any treatment. Presumably part of cancer treatment is nursing care plus all the hideously expensive facilities of our finest hospitals, as well as the expensive services of our finest cancer specialists.

Why in the world should we continue to debate a simple, ridiculously inexpensive adjunct to treatment, like vitamin C, which might, just might, cure the cancer and prevent its return? What earthly reason is there not to at least try it?

In October, 1976 somebody at Associated Press called up the National Cancer Institute in Washington and told them that a physician in Scotland—as we discussed above—had discovered his terminal cancer patients were living four years longer than expected and in reasonably good health when he gave them massive doses of vitamin C. Dr. Linus Pauling was in touch with the doctor and was writing about his work in a number of scientific publications. Was anybody at the National Cancer Institute working on using vitamin C for cancer patients?

Well, yes, he was told by Dr. Paul V. Chretien, chief of Tumor Immunology at the NCI. NCI scientists have given a few healthy people vitamin C for a few days and have found that it stimulates the body's defense systems "and this usually means an increased immune response." We immediately wrote to Dr. Chretien asking for copies of their research papers. We heard nothing from him. In mid-January, 1977, we wrote again and heard nothing from him.

We got in touch with our senators and congressman and asked them if it was possible for them to pry this information out of the National Cancer Institute, since letters from ordinary taxpayers seem to be ignored at the NCI. In due time we got a letter from another NCI scientist enclosing a brief summary of the worldshaking experiment the geniuses at NCI had performed. They had indeed given some vitamin C to five healthy volunteers for a few days and had found that the white blood corpuscles appeared to be in better fighting shape than they had been before the vitamin C. So the cancer specialists came to the conclusion that the vitamin seems to "stimulate the body's defense system." They did not comment on the fact that this stimulation of the body's defense system seems to take place at doses of vitamin C which are quite large—even massive doses. The official recommendation for daily intake of vitamin C is 45 milligrams. The volunteers were given 5,000 to 10,000 milligrams.

So far as we could discover, this is the only bit of research the NCI—supported by millions and millions of dollars of taxpayers' money—has ever done using massive doses of vitamin C to prevent or to treat cancer or even to discover whether there is some slight hope that this harmless vitamin might be effective in preventing this hideous and widespread disease, if given in large enough doses.

Yet in the past NCI scientists have indeed done work along these lines, although it takes a bit of digging to find out about it. In the *Journal of Orthomolecular Psychiatry*, Third Quarter, 1976, Vol. 5, No. 3, Dr. Irwin Stone tells us that in 1969 Dr. Dean Burk and his group at NCI published in the scientific journal *Oncology* (the study of cells) a description of their findings that **vitamin C kills cancer cells and is at the same time harmless to normal cells**.

Their paper began with these words, "The present study shows that ascorbate (vitamin C) is highly toxic or lethal to Ehrlich ascites carcinoma cells in vitro (in a test tube) .... The great advantage that ascorbates possess as potential anticancer agents is that they are, like penicillin, remarkably nontoxic to normal body tissues, and they may be administered to animals in extremely large doses (up to 5 or more grams per kilogram) without notable harmful pharmacological effects."

Dr. Stone comments, "Let me remind you that 5 grams of vitamin C per kilogram for a 150-pound adult amounts to 350 grams or 350,000 milligrams, over three quarters of a pound." The NCI researchers said further that they believed the future of cancer therapy rests not in drugs so toxic that they harm the cancer victim as well as the cancer cells, but in products which are lethal to cancer cells but harmless to healthy cells, like vitamin C.

"They also point out," says Dr. Stone, "that ascorbate was never tested for its anticancer effects by the Cancer

33

Chemotherapy National Service Center because it was too nontoxic to fit into their screening program. They don't want to test anything unless it helps to kill the cancer patient."

Says Dr. Stone, "A substance like ascorbate that will kill cancer cells and be harmless to normal cells has been a long-term goal of cancer researchers, and in 1969 it looked like it had been achieved. One would expect that a crash research program would immediately be organized to check and extend these observations and obtain clinical data on this breakthrough. That was six years ago (eight years ago by now) and no further papers could be found that were published by the NCI on this important subject. Apparently the work was stopped and dropped like a hot potato. If an intensive crash research program had been instituted in 1969, the cancer problem may have been solved by now, or at least we would know a lot more about the role of megascorbate (massive doses of vitamin C) in cancer."

Dr. Stone then describes a case of malignant lymphoma (cancer) in a truck driver treated by Dr. Ewan Cameron in Scotland. The vitamin C treatment was begun only because the orthodox treatment with radiation and drugs was delayed and the man was deteriorating rapidly. He was given 10,000 milligrams of vitamin C intravenously for the first 10 days, then 10,000 milligrams a day by mouth.

The response was so dramatic that the patient said he felt quite well, his appetite returned, his night sweats stopped and he had a general sense of well being. His enlarged liver and spleen returned to normal size and other symptoms of the disease subsided. He went back to work taking 10,000 milligrams of vitamin C daily.

For some unknown reason he stopped taking the vitamin and one month later he was back in the clinic with recurring symptoms. The usual dose of vitamin C failed to bring improvement, the disease progressed and the usual dose of vitamin C did not help. He was then given 20,000 milligrams of the vitamin daily intravenously for two weeks and then 12,500 milligrams daily by mouth thereafter. **"A slow and** sustained clinical improvement was shown and examination about six months later showed him to be normal in all respects," says Dr. Stone. He went back to work, continues to take this large amount of vitamin C every day and has no evidence of active disease.

Dr. Stone tells us that *Medical Tribune* printed in 1954 a case history in which doses up to 42,000 milligrams of vitamin C were given to a victim of **myelogenous leukemia** which gave complete remission of the disease. Every time the vitamin dosage was stopped, as an experiment, the symptoms returned. But within six hours after the victim dosage was started again, the patient improved and remission recurred. "You would think", says Dr. Stone, "that someone in these many years would have tried this harmless megascorbic therapy in the thousands of cases of leukemia that appear each year. A search of the (medical) literature has failed to reveal anyone publishing a check on these exciting clinical results."

Dr. Linus Pauling, speaking before a Biomedical Students Seminar Series at the University of Pennsylvania in February, 1977, said, "A goat the size of a man manufactures (in its liver) 13 grams of vitamin C, or this much," holding up a filled testtube. Holding up another he said, "This one contains the amount a human being manufactures." It was empty. He held up a third, which he said contained 45 milligrams, the amount currently recommended by the Food and Nutrition Board for human adults. The powder appeared as a speck of white at the bottom of the tube. "The Board calls that amount sufficient for 'ordinary good health' but we ought to say 'ordinary poor health'" said Dr. Pauling.

He then attacked the National Cancer Institute for not supporting a study of vitamin C in relation to cancer prevention or treatment. "You know," he said, "the first step in the study of an anti-cancer drug hasn't been carried out for ascorbic acid (vitamin C)—and that is to find out what amount will produce the greatest effect. I'm sure 10 grams is not very optimum."

NCI invited Dr. Pauling to apply for a financial grant to perform animal studies on vitamin C and cancer. He applied for a modest grant five times and was turned down each time because, he was told, *his experiment hadn't been proved!* "Ideas are the rarest commodity in all of science," he said, "and rarest of all at the National Cancer Institute."

In extensive correspondence with the NCI we have never been able to get any satisfactory answer as to why they are determined to ignore the evidence that vitamin C in massive doses might indeed be the answer to cancer therapy and prevention. We can only interpret this as meaning that specialists at NCI, as well as in the many other institutions studying cancer, are protecting their jobs by continuing to tinker with cancer cells and present elaborate theories on the cause of cancer rather than trying the one totally harmless treatment that has been suggested by men of the eminence of Linus Pauling in the scientific world.

The other possible reason is that there is a lot of money to be made producing patented drugs to treat cancer. No one can patent vitamin C, hence there is no money to be made in using it to treat cancer victims.

Dr. Pauling is now working out of The Linus Pauling Institute of Science and Medicine, 2700 Sand Hill Road, Menlo Park, California 94025. They are asking for members and for financial support.

In the meantime, cancer deaths continue to rise.

"Because it strikes young and old alike, because its origins are still so much a mystery and because it is rapidly on the increase, **cancer is the number one health threat confronting our society today,**" according to an article in the Summer, 1976 issue of the *National Resources Defense Council Newsletter.* **"It will kill 370,000 Americans this year (as opposed to about 21,000 in 1918), strike 675,000 others, and cause a loss of over 1,700,000 man-years of potential working life."**

CHAPTER 4

An Incurable
Arthritic Disease
and Vitamin C

ACCORDING TO *The Merck Manual*, 12th Edition, *ankylosing spondylitis* (Marie-Strumpell Disease) is a chronic, progressive disease of the small joints of the spine separable as an entity from rheumatoid arthritis on genetic, epidemiological, pathological, clinical, serologic and therapeutic grounds... neither aspirin nor phenylbutazone (butazolidin) can cure or arrest the progressive ankylosis (stiffness of the spine)."

Statistics reveal that one out of every 330 adult men suffer from *ankylosing spondylitis*. Army doctors have found that it is a frequent cause of backache in soldiers. Also known as *rheumatoid spondylitis*, this disorder especially affects young males, causing complete rigidity of the spine and thorax. The specific cause is not known.

In 1964, Norman Cousins, long-time editor of the prestigious literary magazine, *Saturday Review*, flew home from a lengthy, tiring and frustrating trip abroad. His slight fever and general achiness rapidly developed into a stiff neck and back and great difficulty in moving arms, hand, fingers and legs. His doctor hospitalized him when his sedimentation rate reached 80 mm per hour. The sedimentation rate is the rate at which red blood cells settle out of anticoagulated blood. It may indicate an inflammatory condition, an infection or a cancer.

The doctors decided Mr. Cousins had a very serious collagen disease. This category includes all the arthritic diseases. As the crippling disease progressed, leaving him unable to turn over in bed, the doctors told him he was suffering from *ankylosing spondylitis.* Spondylitis is inflammation of the vertebrae. Ankylosing means stiffening or locking in place. **The patient was faced with eventually being totally unable to move.**

Mr. Cousins' doctors told him he had one chance in 500 of recovering. One specialist said he had never personally seen a recovery from as serious a case as this. Mr. Cousins was being given a number of pain killers for the agonizing pain he was suffering. Associates at the *Saturday Review* researched these drugs and reported to him the highly toxic side effects he might expect. Butazolidin and aspirin were the two he was most worried about, for the doctors prescribed massive doses of both these drugs. A test showed that he was allergic to all of them. He was covered with hives and "felt as though my skin was being chewed up by millions of red ants."

Mr. Cousins decided he would stop using the drugs and somehow get well on his own. His wide reading had acquainted him with many theories on the power of the mind over illness. He knew how terribly destructive to health negative emotions, hopelessness and anxiety can be. He decided he would turn his thoughts to getting well and abandon all negative thinking. He started a program of reading books on humor and laughter and watched comic films sent in by a friend.

Then he remembered his reading about vitamin C. He asked himself, "Couldn't it combat inflammation? Did vitamin C act directly or did it serve as a starter for the body's endocrine (gland) system—in particular, the adrenal glands?

Was it possible, I asked myself, that ascorbic acid had a vital role to play in 'feeding' the adrenal glands?"

He had also read that arthritics seem to be deficient in vitamin C. He thought perhaps this might be because the body uses up its supply of vitamin C in fighting the breakdown of collagen, which is the connective tissue damaged in these diseases. Fortunately his doctor was a long-time friend who had a completely open mind about his treatment and was willing to try anything Cousins suggested.

He told his doctor he wanted to take massive doses of vitamin C. His doctor said he thought there might be danger of kidney damage. Cousins was willing to take the risk. The doctor told him that the largest dose of vitamin C ever given in that hospital was three grams (3,000 milligrams) injected into muscle.

Cousins speculated that "introducing the ascorbic acid directly into the bloodstream might make more efficient use of the vitamin, but I wondered about the body's ability to utilize a sudden massive infusion. **I knew that one of the great advantages of vitamin C is that the body takes only the amount necessary for its purposes and excretes the rest.**... I wondered whether a better procedure than injection would be to administer the ascorbic acid through slow intravenous drip over a period of three or four hours. In this way we could go far beyond the three grams. My hope was to start at 10 grams and then increase the dose daily until we reached 25 grams (25,000 milligrams)."

His doctor was astonished at the suggestion. Again he said he was afraid of kidney damage as well as damage to veins subjected for so long to an intravenous drip. "He said he knew of no data to support the assumption that the body could handle 25 grams over a four-hour period, other than by excreting it rapidly through the urine," says Cousins.

They tested Cousins' blood and started the intravenous drip, administering 10 grams the first day. Within four hours the blood test showed a 9-point improvement.

"Seldom had I known such elation," says Cousins. "The

39

ascorbic acid was working. So was laughter. The combination was cutting heavily into whatever poison was attacking the connective tissue. The fever was receding and the pulse was no longer racing."

They increased the amount of vitamin C a little every day until, by the end of the week, Cousins was getting 25 grams in an intravenous drip. **By this time he was off all drugs and sleeping pills and was sleeping normally.** By the end of the eighth day he was able to move his thumbs without pain. The blood tests continued to improve. Two weeks later he was able to go south to bathe in the warm ocean. He could stand by himself, walk, even jog a bit. For many months he had pain and stiffness when he lifted his arms, his fingers were less skillful than he wished when he played the organ, he sometimes had difficulty turning his head. **But this presumably incurable disease had been conquered without drugs.**

Seven years later, in 1971, he found in *The Lancet*, a British medical journal, **a study of how aspirin destroys vitamin C in the human body. This, apparently, is one reason why arthritics are generally deficient in the vitamin**, since aspirin is the commonest drug used for arthritic pain. "It was no surprise, then," says Cousins, "that I had been able to absorb such massive amounts of ascorbic acid without kidney or other complications."

Norman Cousins' account of his victory over this crippling disease appeared in the conservative *New England Journal of Medicine* for December 23, 1976. In the latter part of his article he speculates on the possibility that vitamin C may have acted as a placebo in his case. A placebo is a pill or treatment which contains nothing of any medicinal value. But often the patient feels better, believing that the pill is powerful. He believed in vitamin C so thoroughly, he says, that perhaps it was his belief rather than any biological action of the vitamin which brought his blood corpuscles back to normal and took the stiffness from his spine. He discusses the place of placebos in medical treatment and suggests that much more research should be done along these lines.

Mr. Cousins describes his visit to the clinic of Dr. Anna Aslan in Rumania who told him she believes there is a direct connection between a strong will to live and chemical balances in the brain. She thinks that the will to live stimulates the entire glandular system, thus possibly bringing about "cures" that are otherwise inexplicable. Of course, Dr. Aslan also uses a drug of the novocaine family which breaks down into a B vitamin inside the body. And she gives immense amounts of tender, loving care, security, hope, encouragement and praise to patients in her geriatric (old folks) clinic.

Dr. F. J. Ingelfinger, the distinguished editor of the *New England Journal of Medicine*, wrote an editorial in the same issue in which the Cousins article appeared, trying to analyze the incident. He reminded his physician readers that miraculous unexplained cures take place sometimes in medicine and that complaints about overwhelming the patient with drugs "are as ancient as the drugs themselves."

"Of greatest interest—at least to me," said Dr. Ingelfinger, "is the nature of Mr. Cousins' processes of reasoning as he cures himself by willpower, laughter, vitamin C and self placebotion . . . here is an astute, perceptive, articulate and distinguished layman who takes his treatment away from the medical establishment and wins out."

How does it happen, then, that his doctors were not as familiar as Mr. Cousins was with the possibility of cure from willpower, laughter and the action of vitamin C, whether real or imagined?

"Well," says Dr. Ingelfinger, "when a patient's condition involves 'a serious collagen illness,' 'adrenal exhaustion,' polypharmacy (lots of drugs), the advantage of a high-fiber diet, and 'allergy tests' for drugs, medical fallibility, perplexity and controversy could hardly be greater; and the latest medical-journal articles on such clinical topics range from pure bunkum to results of experiments that are scientifically unexceptionable but still do no more than

41

nibble away at the margins of vast expanses of ignorance ...at present, it is not possible for the medical establishment, any more than for Mr. Cousins, to speak with confidence about collagen disorders, their protean (variable) manifestations and their often unpredictable course."

We are sorry to say we think this is a cop-out, Dr. Ingelfinger. The incident Mr. Cousins describes happened in 1964. In the ensuing 13 years, so far as we can determine, not a single physician made any attempt to use an intravenous drip of vitamin C for arthritic diseases—whether for its real or imagined value. Mr. Cousins reports no side effects. Such a treatment could have done no harm to the thousands, perhaps hundreds of thousands, of agonized patients who have suffered from this condition in those 13 years. Why has not the medical profession, or the National Institutes of Health, or the Arthritis Foundation, or *somebody in charge of something* experimented further with this harmless therapy, just to see whether they might be able to ease a little pain and stiffness, even if they cannot work the complete miracle Mr. Cousins reports?

Mr. Cousins says he did not make the story public earlier because he did not want to raise false hopes in other sufferers from these diseases. Every treatment given to a victim of a chronic arthritic disease raises false hopes, Mr. Cousins. Aspirin may control the pain for a while. Then the patient can't tolerate any more aspirin. Butazolidin controls the pain but the side effects may be far more devastating than the disease. So the drug must be discontinued. Cortisone, used to ease pain in many other arthritic diseases, is fraught with perils, including the eventual total destruction of the body's bones. Why would it be unethical to "raise false hopes" by giving the patient a completely harmless treatment?

As Mr. Cousins points out plaintively, someone in a hospital is always sticking needles into patients for one purpose or another. Intravenous administration of drugs is quite common. Why, then, not try intravenous administration of a harmless vitamin? We cannot help but feel that the answer has nothing to do with the confusion of the medical profession over methods of treatment of collagen diseases. It has to do rather with the fact that most doctors learn what they know of medical therapy from drug salesmen. No drug salesmen are selling vitamin C. It can't be patented. It costs next to nothing. No money-hungry drug company wants to bother with it. There's more money to be made in new drugs.

Vitamin C is intimately concerned with the manufacture and the health of collagen—the connective tissue which ties all parts of the body together. If you are suffering from one or another of the chronic, extremely painful and disabling collagen (arthritic) diseases, why not show this chapter about Mr. Cousins to your doctor and suggest that he read the original article in the *New England Journal of Medicine*. Do you see any reason for not taking advantage of this therapy, especially if you believe in the helpfulness and beneficence of vitamin C, as Mr. Cousins did?

In the February 18, 1978 issue of the *Saturday Review*, Cousins relates what happened after the article in the *New England Journal of Medicine* was printed. He got letters from 3,000 doctors from about a dozen countries commenting on his *Journal* article. Most of the letters indicated a willingness among doctors to consider new and unconventional approaches to illness.

"There was abundant support for the measures that had figured in my own recovery," says Cousins, "a well developed will to live, laughter and large intravenous doses of sodium ascorbate. Far from resenting the intrusion of a layman into problems of diagnosis and therapy, the doctors who wrote in response to the article warmly endorsed the idea of a patient's partnership with his physician in search of a cure." This certainly seems to be a noble idea for many members of the medical profession to hold.

Two stories from laymen illustrate what happens to most of us when we approach our doctors with suggestions for vitamin therapy. One reader of Cousins' article was a New York lawyer, whose four-year-old daughter was in the hospital with **viral encephalitis**. The doctors had almost nothing to offer in the way of treatment. Cousins told the lawyer he could not, as a layman, give him any advice on medical matters, but he gave him some material from professional journals on the use of vitamin C for treatment of viral diseases.

The lawyer took these to his doctor, who told him he didn't need any medical education from a layman. Certainly he would *not* use vitamin C in treating this child. The lawyer decided on a course of his own. He asked if it was all right for him to give his daughter ice cream when she was able to take it. Of course, he was told. Nothing wrong with ice cream.

The next day the lawyer came to the hospital with a large dish of ice cream spiked with 10 grams (10,000 milligrams) of sodium ascorbate which he fed to his daughter, who ate it eagerly. Sodium ascorbate is a form of vitamin C which is only a bit salty with little of the sourness of ascorbic acid. He gave the child more ice cream with always larger doses of sodium ascorbate every day until she was taking *25 grams daily*, or 25,000 milligrams.

"The lawyer's voice vibrated with elation as he described the child's complete recovery and the prospect of having her home again," says Cousins. "I asked if he had told the specialist what he had done. 'Certainly not,' he replied. 'Why should I make trouble for myself?'"

A letter to Cousins came from a woman whose husband was dying of **cancer**. He had been through surgery, radiation and chemotherapy and she was discouraged at the outlook. Did Cousins think vitamin C might help? Once again, he told her he could give no medical advice, but he sent her material on the work of Dr. Ewan Cameron in Scotland, whose success we discuss in this book.

She asked her doctor (who was a family friend) about using vitamin C. He answered by saying "quack, quack" and raged against such infernal nonsense. She dismissed him, moved her husband out of the hospital and took him home. She started him on vitamin C in large doses and reported to

Cousins that he had gained some ground, that he had a better appetite, had a will to live. "He has already had a few more months of life than seemed possible only a short time ago," she reported.

Some of the doctors who wrote Cousins said it was his faith in his own doctor and his will to live which had saved him. **Others said it was the vitamin C, and they told many stories of their own work with this vitamin which is, apparently, harmless in doses that are astronomically high.**

Two Illinois scientists sent him information on their work showing the essential nature of vitamin C in regard to an enzyme which is responsible for the health of collagen, the very material of which we are made—the substance that breaks down in the arthritic diseases.

Cousins points out that **in many British hospitals it is now common practice to give intravenous doses of vitamin C before surgery, rather than giving antibiotics.** Dr. Cameron, the Scots physician who treats cancer with vitamin C, says that a certain enzyme—hyaluronidase—attacks collagen which is the intercellular cement. So long as this enzyme is free to attack cellular material, just so long can cancer cells proliferate. Proliferation will stop when the release of this enzyme stops. **Vitamin C strengthens the basic material of which collagen is made, so it stops the proliferation of cancer cells.** And it is this terrible proliferation which eventually destroys cancer victims.

Then years after his sojourn in the hospital with an "incurable" arthritic disease, Cousins met on the street in New York one of the specialists who had given him no hope of recovery. Cousins gave the doctor a handshake that caused the physician to wince and plead for release. He said, "I see you're well. How did you do it?"

It is noteworthy that Norman Cousins gives a great deal of credit for his recovery to his wife who, he says, has a positive outlook on life and "believes deeply in the advantages of good nutrition."

He also says that, "Hundreds of letters from doctors ... reflected the view that no medication they could give their patients is as potent as the state of mind that a patient brings to his or her own illness. In this sense, they said, the most valuable service a physician can provide to a patient is helping him mobilize all the resources of mind and body in order to maximize his own recuperative and healing potentialities."

We think this important article may mark a turning point in the attitude of the medical progression in general in regard to vitamin therapy for preventing and treating illnesses. As this is being written, in March, 1978, a World Congress on Vitamin C is being held in California, attended by professional people—scientists, physicians and psychiatrists—from all over the world. No doubt the testimony on significant and valuable work being done with this vitamin will get publicity not only in medical and scientific journals, but also in newspapers and magazines of general circulation. The Congress was also commemorating the 50th anniversary of the discovery of vitamin C. One of the participants was its discoverer, Dr. Albert Szent-Gyorgyi.

CHAPTER 5

Try to Prevent
a Cold

"Do you know what it is to succumb under an insurmountable day-mare—a 'whoreson lethargy,' Falstaff calls it—an indisposition to do anything or to be anything; a total deadness and distaste; a suspension of vitality; an indifference to locality; a numb, soporifical good-for-nothingness; an ossification all over; an oysterlike insensibility to the passing events; a mind-stupor; a brawny defiance to the needles of a thrusting-in conscience? Did you ever have a very bad cold...?

"I am weary of the world; life is weary of me. My day has gone into twilight, and I don't think it worth the expense of candles.... I inhale suffocation. I can't distinguish veal from mutton; nothing interests me.... If you told me the world will be at an end tomorrow, I should say, 'Will it?' I have not volition enough left to dot my eyes, much less to comb my eyebrows; my eyes are set in my head; my brains are gone out to see a poor relation in Moorfields and they did not say when they'd come back again... my hand writes, not I, from habit, as chickens run about a little when their heads are off....

"Did you ever have an obstinate cold—six or seven weeks' unremitting chill and suspension of hope, fear, conscience and everything? Yet do I try all I can to cure it; I try wine and

47

spirits and smoking and snuff, in unsparing quantities; but they all only seem to make me worse instead of better .... Who shall deliver me from the body of this death?"

These dreary words were written to a friend in 1824 by the famous English essayist, Charles Lamb. In those days, as you see, one tried to cure colds with wine and whisky, smoking and snuff. **As we know today, colds are caused by 70 to 80 varieties of viruses.** Doctors have no drug that kills cold viruses, so it seems futile to go to a doctor for treatment of a cold. Nevertheless, most doctors give cold victims some antibiotics which may help them to avoid aftermaths of a cold which are often caused by bacteria rather than viruses.

Aside from this, we are, like Charles Lamb, faced with just suffering through the cold and whatever follows it, unless we have been wise enough to prepare for the cold season long before it arrives. How do you do this? **Foreign invaders of the body are fought by white blood cells.** They are the soldiers provided by the body to surround the invader and engulf it. They form a circle around the bacteria or virus and simply overwhelm it and destroy it.

So it would seem very sensible to coddle these white blood cells and make sure they are present in large numbers by the time the cold season is here. **They are made of protein.** The body cannot manufacture them of fat or carbohydrate. This is believed to be **one of the main reasons why people suffering from deficiency in protein are so easily susceptible to infections.** They do not have enough white blood cells in good condition to fight off the infection agents.

How much protein are you getting on a year-round basis? High protein foods are all those of animal origin—meat, fish, poultry, eggs and dairy products, plus all those seed foods like wholegrains, nuts, soybeans, lentils, sunflower and squash seeds. When we say "meat" is the best source of protein we do not mean just "beef." All meat, as well as all fish and poultry, contain about the same amount of protein, so there is no need to stuff yourself with expensive steak in the

48

mistaken notion that this is what is meant by protein. Seek out lean meats, for, of course, the less fat the meat contains, the more protein it contains. We tend to eat too much fat.

Vegetable sources of protein are the wholegrain, unprocessed kind. The wholegrain cereals at your health food store contain far more protein than the sugary ones at the supermarket. Wheat germ and wheat bran are two of the very best sources of dietary protein. Unprocessed seeds like peanuts and sunflower seeds are loaded with protein, along with B vitamins, many minerals and a lot of fiber which is important to good health.

The other nutrient which is present in large amounts in the protective white blood cells is vitamin C. It is also stored in the adrenal glands which help us to endure stress. This suggests that vitamin C plays a very important role in protecting us from colds. And in preventing colds. The only animals which get colds are human beings and apes. These are also almost the only living things which do not manufacture their own vitamin C.

Irwin Stone tells us in his fine book, *The Healing Factor— Vitamin C Against Disease*—that scientists have known since vitamin C was discovered that it has a powerful effect on viruses. Early researchers tested it against viruses of polio, vaccinia, herpes, rabies, foot-and-mouth disease and a plant disease, tobacco mosaic, and found that the vitamin destroys the viruses speedily. By 1939, one worker in this field prophesied that **"Vitamin C may truthfully be designated as the 'antitoxic' and 'antiviral' vitamin."**

Dr. Stone recounts early attempts to stop or cure colds using very small doses of the vitamin—up to 300 milligrams a day. No spectacular results were achieved, although people who got even this much vitamin C were spared the frequent aftermath of tonsilitis—rheumatic fever and pneumonia. In 1948, a physician injected 450 milligrams of vitamin C immediately after the onset of a cold. By injecting the vitamin he got quicker and more effective results. Half of his patients were completely relieved, usually after the first or second injection. In 2,000 injections there were no complications. Says Stone, "an astronomical number of colds could have been prevented in the intervening years if only this early work had been followed up."

A number of other scientists and physicians, using large doses, gave very favorable reports during the following years. **By 1958, H. Miegl reported excellent results using 2 to 5 grams (2,000 to 5,000 milligrams) of vitamin C for respiratory diseases, nosebleeds, radiation sickness, postoperative bleeding and other conditions.**

N. W. Markwell in 1947 used three-fourths of a gram of vitamin C or more every three or four hours and said, "My experience seems to show that **if the dose is given both early enough and in large enough quantity, the chances of stopping a cold are about fifty-fifty, or perhaps better**. It is an amazing and comforting experience to realize suddenly in the middle of the afternoon that no cold is present, after having in the morning expected several days of throat torture.... **I have never seen any ill effects whatsoever from vitamin C and I do not think there are any....**"

Dr. Stone recommends the following preventive therapy for colds. First of all, he thinks all of us should be taking up to 5 grams of vitamin C daily (5,000 milligrams). He says that anyone who does will have a high resistance to respiratory diseases. "Should the exposure to the infectious agent be unduly heavy or some other uncorrected biochemical stresses be imposed, the infecting virus may gain a foothold and start developing . . . it is much easier to abort an incipient cold than to try to treat an advanced case. If a known heavy exposure to the infectious agent is experienced, such as close contacts with a coughing and sneezing cold sufferer, then extra prophylactic (preventive) doses of several grams of ascorbic acid (vitamin C), several times a day may be taken without waiting for cold symptoms to develop.

"At the first symptoms of a developing cold, I take about

1.5 to 2 grams of ascorbic acid. Within twenty minutes to half an hour another dose is ingested and this is repeated at 20 minute to half hour intervals. Usually by the third dose, the virus has been effectively inactivated, and usually no further cold symptoms will appear. I watch for any delayed symptoms and, if any become evident, I take further doses. If the start of the regimen is delayed and it is instituted only after the virus has spread throughout the body, the results may not be so dramatic, but ascorbic acid will nevertheless be of great benefit."

Dr. Linus Pauling, the two-time Nobel Prize winner, became interested in Dr. Stone's research and wrote *Vitamin C and the Common Cold*, which plunged this distinguished scientist into a vortex of scientific controversy, during which he was called every insulting name his enemies could devise. Throughout the attacks, Pauling and Stone have continued to write about and champion vitamin C for maintaining good health and for preventing the common cold.

Poor Charles Lamb, suffering through a bleak English winter with his seven weeks of cold symptoms, knew so little of how to maintain good health that he tried to cure his cold with alcoholic beverages and smoking. Vitamins were not discovered until almost 100 years later. **There is no way to know how the history of the world might have changed had vitamin C been available in large doses down through the ages.** Could widespread plagues and infectious diseases of all kinds have been prevented? We do not know. It seems possible.

It also seems possible that **we could wipe out the common cold in a matter of years by simply seeing to it that everyone gets enough vitamin C** throughout the year to protect him from the first symptoms of a cold. And if a cold should creep up on him unaware, chances are very good that vitamin C can conquer it.

CHAPTER 6

Vitamin C for Drug Addicts

AN INNOVATIVE APPROACH to treating drug addicts is discussed at length by Drs. Alfred F. Libby and Irwin Stone in a paper, "The Hypoascorbemia-Kwashiorkor Approach to Drug Addiction Therapy. A Pilot Study." The paper was read at a meeting of the Western Regional Seminar of the International Academy of Preventive Medicine, and it was to be published in the *Journal of Orthomolecular Psychiatry*.

To translate, *Hypoascorbemia* is the name that Dr. Stone has given to the condition in which all human beings live—a lack of enough vitamin C for perfect health because they have lost the ability to manufacture this substance in their livers, as practically all other animals do. The word means "too little ascorbic acid" (vitamin C).

Kwashiorkor is the unpronounceable word referring to a nutritional condition most often found among infants and young children in the tropics and subtropics, occurring soon after weaning, due primarily to not enough high quality protein. The symptoms of this dietary deficiency disease are edema (swelling), skin changes, impaired growth, fatty liver and severe apathy and weakness.

Drs. Libby and Stone have found that drug addiction produces in its victims severe scurvy—the

disease of vitamin C deficiency—along with many other deficiencies in various vitamins and minerals and in high quality protein.

A memo from Dr. Stone summarizing the article mentioned above tells us that the Methadone program for "treating" these sick people merely substitutes a legal narcotic for an illegal one. This just continues the severe biochemical stress contributing to their illness.

So Drs. Stone and Libby decided to try nutritional therapy. They named the condition of the drug addicts Hypoascorbemia-Kwashiorkor—that is, too little vitamin C and too little high quality protein. They treated both the lack of vitamin C and lack of all the various nutritional elements involved in the deficiency disease from which these addicts appear to be suffering.

They tell us that the treatment is inexpensive, non-toxic, uses no drugs or narcotics and is entirely "orthomolecular," a word coined by Dr. Linus Pauling to mean supplying to the body the optimum amount of nutritional material, especially substances normally present in the human body, rather than drugs. Such substances include, of course, vitamins, minerals and high quality protein. **Drs. Stone and Libby tell us their treatment was rapidly effective in bringing good health to the addicts they treated.**

They began with immense doses of ascorbic acid in the form of sodium ascorbate—25 to 85 grams a day (20,000 to 85,000 milligrams) along with massive doses of other vitamins, minerals and protein in an easily assimilated form. Under this treatment, they say, the heroin or Methadone is stopped and no withdrawal symptoms are encountered. If the addict takes a "fix," it is immediately detoxified and no "high" is produced. It is like injection of plain water.

There is great improvement in well being and mental alertness among the addicts. In a few days, say the two California scientists, appetite returns and they eat well. They have restful sleep and the constipation which Methadone brings is relieved. After about four to six days, the dosages are reduced to "holding levels."

In 30 addicts tested in this pilot study the results were excellent in all cases. It appears that this simple, non-toxic inexpensive procedure should serve as the basis for large-scale testing to develop a new program for freeing drug addicts from their addiction.

In drug overdosage, sodium ascorbate can be a life-saving measure, they tell us. Unconscious over-dosed addicts are given the sodium ascorbate intravenously, 30 to 50 grams, while those able to swallow can be given the same quantity in a glass of milk. (Sodium ascorbate does not have the sharp acid taste of ascorbic acid. It has a faint salty taste, nothing more).

This antidote is non-specific, say the scientists, and works on all drugs, so no time need be wasted in identifying the drug. "We speculate on ascorbate's action as due to the high levels of sodium ascorbate in the brain as competing for and displacing the narcotic from the opiate receptor sites. If this be the case, then it might be possible to use this phenomenon post-operatively on surgical patients to quickly bring them out of anesthesia," Drs. Libby and Stone say.

They go on to tell the physicians and psychiatrists who will be reading their article in the professional journal just where and how to get the vitamins they used and in what form and potency they are available.

We think this information is world-shaking. If one adds up all the misery involved in drug addiction: the suffering, the degradation, the crime, the jail sentences, the destruction of careers, families and personality, it is difficult to think of anything that holds greater promise for the world than this harmless, inexpensive treatment which would bring the addict back to health without withdrawal symptoms and give him or her the chance to start a new life, well buttressed with nutritional aid that practically guarantees no return to a drug-oriented life. **For the person who is well nourished—truly well nourished—has no need for drugs, does not feel any craving for them.**

Perhaps best of all is the fact that the former addict will be able to take his "medicine" home with him and will not have to depend on visits to his doctor's office. The "medicine" consists only of harmless vitamins, minerals and protein. And so long as he or she takes them and sticks to a good, nourishing diet at mealtime there seems to be little chance that a return to addiction should occur.

Professional readers can address their requests for reprints of the *Journal* article to Dr. Alfred F. Libby, 520 West 17th St., Santa Ana, California 92706. For others, the material is too technical to be of any use.

CHAPTER 7

What Causes
Crib Death?

WE RECENTLY LISTENED to the tape of an Australian radio program on the subject of infant and baby health. The chief topic under discussion was Sudden Infant Death (SID) or, as it is called by laymen in our country, Crib Death. This is the terrible fate of a happy, apparently healthy baby put to bed by his mother, only to be found dead or near death when she looks in to check on him later.

There are many theories as to the cause of Crib Death. Its victims are not only the babies, but parents and other relatives as well, who may go into serious depression, complete mental breakdown or lifelong guilt complexes, haunted by the thought that the baby's death may be somehow their fault. It happens perhaps up to 20,000 times a year in the United States and just as frequently in other countries.

One theory holds that **bottle-fed children are more susceptible to Crib Death than breast-fed ones** because mother's milk provides antibodies which protect her nursing child from many kinds of infection. (Many of the children who die from Crib Death are known to have had slight respiratory infections at the time). How, then, does it happen that breast-fed children also succumb to Crib Death?

The doctors who spoke in Australia believe that **lack of vitamin C may be largely responsible for Crib Death**, combined with the extra stress on the child from the numerous immunizations which are customarily given very young infants. Dr. Archie Kalokerinos told of Aborigine babies in the Australian areas where he practices medicine. He was horrified when he came to the area to discover that **one out of every two Aborigine babies was dying from unknown causes very early in life**. All the babies and children brought to him suffered almost constantly from runny noses, infected ears and coughs. Gastrointestinal diseases and pneumonia were commonplace. They occurred in the same children. It was evident that the children were badly nourished and lived under unhygienic conditions. So Dr. Kalokerinos gave them antibiotics and the customary vitamin supplements.

He says, in his startling book on the subject, *Every Second Child*, "If it was known that the diet included, for example, 30 milligrams of vitamin C...a day then there seemed no reason for concern...Much had been written about this vital subject and an enormous amount of research had been done. One leading research institute after another had clearly demonstrated that under conditions of stress, infections and injury there was an increased utilization of vitamin C and 30 milligrams a day may not be sufficient to cope with the increased demand." But this information had been ignored by the medical profession and even dedicated physicians like Dr. Kalokerinos had not heard of this research.

When he did hear about it, **Dr. Kalokerinos brought these tragic figures on child mortality down to zero by simply giving all the babies who were brought to him enough vitamin C** to prevent any deficiency, no matter how great was the stress to which the child was exposed and how great the child's need for the vitamin. The photographs in his book show babies brought in with tender limbs, irritability, "running" ears, teething problems—all desperately needing much more vitamin C than they had been getting. And there

57

are pictures of the babies relaxed, sleepy and smiling after injections of vitamin C.

Speaking of SID deaths, Dr. Kalokerinos says, "Some sudden unexpected deaths occur in infants who appear to be perfectly well, do not suffer from illnesses of any sort, are placed in a cot to rest or sleep and are later found dead. Mostly no cause is found and these are typical cases. I hesitate before stating that all these typical cases are due to vitamin C deficiency. Some definitely are. It is possible that they all are... often death is not really sudden. An infant may appear to be mildly ill, then suddenly collapse, become shocked and die. The variation of the infant's requirements for vitamin C are tremendous. Adults do not exhibit this. Adult scurvy is therefore a slow process."

One possible cause of the baby's greatly increased need for vitamin C is the immunization program which, in Australia as in our country, is almost mandatory for very young infants. Dr. Kalokerinos noticed that Crib Deaths and other unexplained deaths were more frequent in winter (when fresh foods rich in vitamin C were unavailable) and during and after immunization programs. There seems to be no doubt that immunization for childhood diseases is a form of great stress. This means that the baby's need for vitamin C increases greatly. If no provision is made for this by increasing the baby's intake of vitamin C, a condition resembling scurvy or scurvy itself will probably follow.

Many of the children Dr. Kalokerinos treated had no visible symptoms of vitamin C deficiency. Others had the aching bones, the irritability, the swollen gums which any old-time doctor would have recognized as scurvy. But modern physicians have been convinced that all babies get plenty of vitamin C in their formulas or in fruit juice, so they do not anticipate any scurvy symptoms nor look for them.

Dr. Fred Klenner of North Carolina, who uses massive doses of vitamin C to treat many disorders, spoke on the Australian radio program. He is a specialist in chest and respiratory diseases. **He said that any child with nasal**

congestion is a likely candidate for Crib Death. He gives all infants and children in his care up to one gram (1,000 milligrams) of vitamin C daily. He said that any doctor who tries it will discover that **vitamin C, in proper amounts, will destroy a virus within 96 minutes or less, especially if the vitamin is injected.** Victims of Crib Death die from suffocation, he said. He prescribes one-half to one gram of vitamin C every hour, if the child with a respiratory disease has a temperature less than 100 degrees. If it is over that, he gives the vitamin by injection.

Mothers ask him why babies die in bed rather than during the day. They are put to bed with stuffed nostrils, he says, resulting from respiratory infections, however slight. They die of suffocation. By destroying the infectious virus you prevent the nasal stuffiness. Mothers should also clean mucus from any infant's nostrils very carefully before putting the child to bed, if any evidence of colds or nasal stuffiness is present.

Other physicians on the program told of finding many infants with no vitamin C at all in their urine. One doctor said that one mother out of every 24 that he treats has no vitamin C in her breast milk. Australian babies are given a formula called "Sunshine milk" which contains no vitamin C. If babies of mothers who are also deficient in vitamin C are given no vitamin supplements containing this essential substance they will surely suffer from lack of the vitamin which is used in many body processes, which is easily and rapidly excreted and easily destroyed by many toxins.

Cigarette smoke, for example. **The prospective mother who smokes will surely have no vitamin C to pass along to her unborn baby since smoking destroys vitamin C in our bodies.** The child who grows up in a house where the air is thick with cigarette smoke is getting almost as much exposure to the toxin as adults are, and, since he is so much smaller, the effects on him are probably much more serious.

"125 Crib Death infants, followed from birth, were compared to a similar group of living babies," says *American*

Journal of Diseases of Children, November, 1976. "Some of the Crib Death victims showed evidence of brain dysfunction including abnormalities in breathing, feeding and temperature regulation. **More of the dead infants had been born to mothers who smoked and had anemia.**"

Homeostasis Quarterly is published by the Adrenal Metabolic Research Society of the Hypoglycemia Foundation. Its Summer, 1975 issue dealt with Crib Death. Here is a quote:

"*The New York Times*, July 5, 1975 carried a report on the findings of Dr. Henry Lardy, Wisconsin University Enzyme Institute, pointing to a defect in amino acid (protein) metabolism with resulting low blood sugar levels, as a possible cause of sudden infant death. Dr. Lardy observed, if a baby's ability to synthesize sugar is not efficient, as long as he is fed every few hours, he is fine. However, during a long fast, sleeping through the night, for instance, or missing a feeding, the blood sugar may fall extremely low and the baby may not be able to convert amino acids efficiently with resulting fatal hypoglycemia (low blood sugar). It was pointed out, in addition, that **a number of babies, victims of SID, had a history of 'fits' and fits are a classic symptom of low blood sugar.** Dr. Lardy presented his report at the First Annual Workshop on Sudden Infant Death Syndrome, sponsored by the National Institutes of Health.

"Sudden Infant Death Syndrome is a tragic situation, one which is well understood by the editor of *Homeostasis*, who lost her only child in this fashion 18 years ago. Numbers of theories have been put forward as to the cause. Now there is a breakthrough. Inefficient blood sugar regulation dominates the scene. Pertinent is a report on clinical aspects of hypoglycemia in newborn infants (Fluge, G., *Acta Paediat. Scand.* 63:826, 1974). Dr. Fluge stresses the need for blood glucose (sugar) determination in ALL infants, pointing out those at particular risk are infants born to mothers who had toxemia of pregnancy and infants, full-term, but low birth weight." For a copy of this very significant article in full, write to the Society named above at P.O. Box 98, Fleetwood, Mount Vernon, New York 10552. And send along a donation to help Mrs. Marilyn Hamilton Light in her important work.

There is also research to show that lack of vitamin E may be a contributing cause of Crib Death. British physicians tell us that babies are born with much lower levels of vitamin E in their blood than adults have. As a result they may develop a kind of anemia which is treated by giving them vitamin E. Levels of vitamin E in blood rise much more slowly in babies given formulas than in those who are breast-fed. Studies of victims of Crib Death indicate that levels of this vitamin are lower in their blood than in the blood of normal infants. Animals on diets deficient in vitamin E show many of the complications Crib Death victims show when they are autopsied. Tests of the infant formulas now on sale in our country have shown that they contain almost no vitamin E and are high in polyunsaturated fats which increase the body's need for this vitamin.

A new book on *Crib Death* by Richard H. Raring discusses just about everything that is known officially about this epidemic disaster, including a chapter on "Theories and Research", in which he touches on the subject of vitamins and other diet deficiencies. Mr. Raring had apparently not heard of the Australian research when he wrote his book, for he dismisses Dr. Klenner's use of vitamin C in massive doses as "one more theory, neither proven, disproven nor tested."

This brings us to a realization of the fact that Crib Death, like cancer, may have a multitude of manifestations and a multitude of causes. So far orthodox medical science has turned up nothing which gives parents any hope that their baby can escape this terrible fate. It seems to us that any intelligent parent, faced with the facts, must realize that giving vitamins to a baby is no more difficult and no more risky than giving him food and water. So why quibble about whether the "theories" on low blood sugar, vitamin C and vitamin E are just "theories" or whether they can be useful in preventing this tragedy? Let the scientists and researchers quibble and nitpick! They go through this procedure with every new idea that appears in the realm of health, disease and medicine, especially if vitamins are involved. But, meanwhile, give your baby whatever chance for a healthy life you can give him by using whatever helpful information you can find—including the well-documented facts from Dr. Kalokerinos and Dr. Klenner as well as the article in *Homeostasis*. The cost is pennies. You may be buying health and safety for your baby. Why wait?

The books referred to above are:

Every Second Child, by Archie Kalokerinos, available from the Book Department at Bronson Pharmaceuticals, 2546 Rinetti Lane, La Canada, California 91011. Price, $8.10.

Crib Death, by Richard H. Raring, published by Exposition Press, Inc., 900 South Oyster Bay Road, Hicksville, New York 11901 for $6.50.

CHAPTER 8

Vitamin C
May Lower
Cholesterol Levels

MEDICAL EVIDENCE is rapidly accumulating that **vitamin C may be a powerful agent in lowering blood cholesterol and preventing the hardening of the arteries** that often results following such high levels of the fatty substance.

Medical World News for September 13, 1974 told the story of a British physician's observations and experiments in relation to vitamin C. Dr. Constance Spittle is consultant pathologist at the Pinderlands General Hospital in Wakefield, England. **Dr. Spittle believes that hardening of the arteries is a disease of vitamin C deficiency.** She also believes that getting large doses of **the vitamin may help to prevent deep vein thrombosis**—the crisis that so often follows major surgery.

Dr. Spittle started her research on vitamin C during a period when she was experimenting with a diet consisting of nothing but fresh fruits and vegetables. The diet failed utterly to sustain her and she had to give it up, but she discovered, while she was on the diet, that the levels of cholesterol in her blood declined from 240 milligrams percent to 160 milligrams percent at the end of her experiment.

She thought this must be the result of a diet in which there was no cholesterol, for completely vegetarian foods do not contain this fatty substance. But after she returned to her former diet, her cholesterol levels continued to decline. She added large amounts of fresh fruits and vegetables to her diet. The cholesterol levels continued to decline. Then she boiled all the fruits and vegetables thoroughly before eating them. The cholesterol levels began to climb once again. Apparently something essential was destroyed in the boiling process. Could it be vitamin C? It is well known that the vitamin is destroyed when fresh foods are cooked too long.

She persuaded some of her colleagues to try an experiment. She gave them one gram (1,000 milligrams) of vitamin C daily for six weeks and took regular measurements of their cholesterol levels. In some the levels dropped. In others they were increased. She had begun to suspect that vitamin C might be related to preventing the plaques that appear on the inside of blood vessels and produce hardening of the arteries. So she gave vitamin C to 25 patients with hardening of the arteries. In some of them the cholesterol levels went up. In others they dropped.

But it seemed that the lower cholesterol levels occurred in young people. They rose in older people, especially those suffering from hardening of the arteries. Dr. Spittle believes there is a good reason for this. Vitamin C, she says, has the job of collecting the cholesterol in arteries and transporting it to the liver where it is transformed into certain digestive juices which help to digest fats.

In young people, says Dr. Spittle, where there is little cholesterol in their arteries, there is a net flow from the blood to the liver. But in older people whose arteries are more "furred," or lined, with cholesterol deposits, the vitamin C pulls out more cholesterol from the arteries than it can readily transport to the liver, so the blood levels go up. In those with fully developed hardening of the arteries, the situation is worst.

But eventually the vitamin C will transport this unwanted cholesterol to the liver and this will produce an improvement in the condition of the patient, says Dr. Spittle. She says that many of the patients who suffered from hardening of the arteries told her they felt better during the experiment. They could walk farther without pain or breathlessness. Dr. Spittle says it is futile just to study the *levels* of cholesterol in blood.

Instead, she says, doctors should study what effects the vitamin C has on the levels. If it pushes them up, then probably the patient was suffering from hardening of the arteries, but the vitamin sent the offending cholesterol on its way to the liver. This means everything should proceed on its normal course. **The vitamin C appears to have the important function of loosening cholesterol from artery walls and sending it along to the liver,** as well as taking part in the changes that take place in the liver.

But Dr. Spittle also believes that lack of vitamin C may be responsible for starting the whole process of artery hardening to begin with. Plaques of cholesterol form on damaged places in the inner wall of the artery. If this original damage could be prevented, hardening of the arteries might be prevented.

Dr. Spittle believes that vitamin C can and does prevent such damage. Vitamin C is involved in the manufacture of the "cement" or "glue" that holds cells together. This is especially important in the cells that line the arteries. If one is deficient in vitamin C, damaged parts heal slowly and plaques may appear. When there is plenty of vitamin C around, healing is rapid and cholesterol deposits are prevented.

To test her theories on human arteries would require a lifetime, for the individuals tested would have to grow old during the test. So Dr. Spittle is now working on a theory regarding deep vein thrombosis. This is the blood clot that so often forms after surgery when a blood clot snags on the damaged part of a vein.

Using 60 surgery patients as subjects, Dr. Spittle gave 30 of them one gram (1,000 milligrams) of vitamin C daily, while the other 30 received a tablet containing nothing. The number of clots in patients taking the vitamin was only half the expected number and these were so minor they could barely be detected. Many surgeons in Dr. Spittle's hospital are now routinely giving their patients vitamin C after surgery, with good results.

In this same hospital **the section for treatment of burns has been giving large amounts of vitamin C for six years**, to hasten healing. During that time there was only one fatal lung clot and no deep vein thrombosis—"an achievement far outstripping that seen in other similar units not using vitamin C."

So it seems that by keeping cholesterol moving in the right direction—toward the liver—and by functioning correctly with it, after it arrives in the liver, **vitamin C may perhaps prevent hardening of the arteries, keeping the insides of arteries clean and free from plaques or clots.** For people with suspected hardening of the arteries, Dr. Spittle recommends one gram of vitamin C daily. She takes half a gram with breakfast and eats a lot of fresh fruits and vegetables—all raw, so that their abundant vitamin C content is preserved.

As if to confirm directly Dr. Spittle's research comes word from Bratislava, Czechoslovakia, that **Dr. Emil Ginter has reduced high cholesterol levels in middle-aged men and women by giving them 300 milligrams of vitamin C daily**. These people were admittedly short on the vitamin because it was during that season of the year when fresh foods were scarce.

At the Institute of Human Research, Dr. Ginter gave the vitamin for 47 days to people chronically short on vitamin C and chronically found to have high cholesterol levels. These levels dropped an average of 33 milligrams percent in 13 subjects. The reactions were most dramatic in those whose cholesterol levels were highest.

In more recent trials, 1,000 milligrams of vitamin C daily decreased blood levels of triglycerides—another worrisome kind of fatty substance often found in quantity where hardening of the arteries threatens. In patients with the highest levels of this fat, a measurement of 308 milligrams percent dropped to 197 milligrams. In those with slightly lower levels an average of 262 milligrams dropped to 236 milligrams.

In his earlier studies with guinea pigs—almost the only animals aside from human beings which do not manufacture their own vitamin C—Dr. Ginter had produced swelling of the inner walls of the arteries and other symptoms of artery disease by depriving the animals of vitamin C for long periods of time. He did not reduce their vitamin C intake low enough for the animals to get scurvy, but just enough to leave them in a subclinical state of scurvy, which many scientists believe may be the situation many human beings find themselves in these days. These animals, too, had raised levels of cholesterol in their blood and in their livers.

Dr. Ginter believes that vitamin C is necessary for processing cholesterol into digestive juices, which is its normal fate in the liver. If there is not enough vitamin C, this process does not go smoothly. Along with Dr. Spittle, Dr. Ginter believes that disorders of fat metabolism and disorders in the wall of the artery and disorders in the coagulating ability of the blood may all be associated with lack of vitamin C and all may contribute to the final problem which is hardening of the arteries and, possibly, eventual heart attacks or strokes.

"There is now substantial evidence that chronic latent scurvy is prevalent in man," say three Australian physicians. Scurvy is the disease of vitamin C deficiency. By "chronic" and "latent" these doctors mean that, while people are not dying in an epidemic of scurvy as they did many years ago, before anyone knew what caused this disease, still there is substantial evidence that most of us are suffering all the time from just getting not enough vitamin C.

Writing in the medical publication *Atherosclerosis* (Volume 24, 1976), these doctors state that evidence for **the benefits of reducing hardening of the arteries by vitamin C appears to be as strong right now as was the evidence in the early 1950s for the benefits of polyunsaturated fats**, which doctors believed would reduce cholesterol in the blood and thus prevent hardening of the arteries.

But now, according to Dr. S. D. Turley, C. E. West and B. J. Horton of the Australian National University, we know that trials with salad oils and margarines have not produced conclusive results showing that they will reduce cholesterol in blood or that reducing cholesterol in blood will prevent heart attacks. What we need now, they say, are experiments or observations on a large number of people to test the effectiveness of vitamin C in reducing deaths from heart disease.

We have had evidence since 1940, they go on, indicating that **blood cholesterol levels can be lowered in those people in whom they are too high by giving them vitamin C**. Since then, a number of researchers have done tests which have produced conflicting results. We are quite sure that many people—especially older folks and younger people living in institutions are not getting nearly enough vitamin C to remain healthy, so they suffer from "subclinical scurvy."

Only in recent years have scientists used guinea pigs with subclinical scurvy to test their theories on hardening of the arteries and heart attacks. As we mentioned, guinea pigs and human beings are among the few which do not make their own vitamin C in the liver. Before this, scientists made the mistake of using animals like rats which make their own vitamin C, or they used guinea pigs with a fullblown case of scurvy. Neither of these animals is in the condition that most human beings are in—subclinical scurvy.

Research done correctly seems to show that **deficiency in vitamin C may contribute to hardening of the**

arteries and heart attacks in two ways. First, the vitamin may actually regulate the amount of fatty material in the blood, thus preventing build-up of fats on the interior walls of arteries. Then, too, the vitamin may also protect against hardening of the arteries by nourishing the arteries and not allowing the build-up of fats and minerals on their inner walls.

Most studies have shown, say the Australian doctors, that **vitamin C deficiency leads to high cholesterol levels in blood and unnatural accumulation of cholesterol in other tissues, as well.** Most studies have shown that animals with the least vitamin C in their tissues have the most serious symptoms of hardening of the arteries. And it seems true, as well, that giving plenty of vitamin C to animals and to people with high cholesterol levels will reduce those levels.

Scientists do not as yet understand just how vitamin C reduces cholesterol levels. Probably, they think, it has to do with reducing the manufacture of a digestive juice, hence slowing down the absorption of cholesterol from food. **Getting plenty of vitamin C also lowers the amount of triglycerides in blood.** Some specialists believe that high triglyceride levels are much more dangerous than high cholesterol levels.

Unfortunately, these Australian doctors do not carry their ideas to the conclusion which it seems to us is necessary. They claim that there is no need to take very large doses of vitamin C. Just enough to bring daily vitamin C intake up to the recommended allowance will do, they believe. We don't know how they arrived at this conclusion, especially since, in our country at least, there is little doubt that many of the people who are dying from heart attacks are well-to-do, knowledgeable people who certainly get their orange juice every morning, eat their salad at lunch and probably take a one-a-day vitamin pill with maybe 50 to 100 milligrams of vitamin C in it. That brings their vitamin C intake well above the officially recommended amount of 45 milligrams. Why, then, are such people dying in an epidemic of heart attacks?

Perhaps it might be because many of them smoke. **Cigarette smoke destroys vitamin C wholesale in a laboratory testtube and in human blood.** Dr. Irwin Stone, who has devoted himself to the study of vitamin C for many years, believes that the average human being who is not under stress needs as much as 5 to 20 grams (5,000 to 20,000 milligrams) of vitamin C daily and a smoker should take 3 to 5 grams more than that for every pack of cigarettes smoked. If smoking were the only stress to which such people are exposed, this might be enough. But there are other stresses. Every new stress makes demands on body stores of vitamin C.

Carbon monoxide and other elements in air pollution, for example. Chemicals in food and water. Drugs. Almost everybody these days is taking a prescription drug or an over-the-counter drug with no knowledge of how much vitamin C might be destroyed in the body by this drug. Stress itself greatly increases our need for vitamin C—the stress of work, of commuting, of family and job problems, the tension produced by crowds, noise and frustration.

It seems to us that it's the combined total of all these stresses which makes our need for vitamin C far, far greater than the amount needed to protect us from subclinical scurvy. What we want is superlative health. Getting enough vitamin C is one way to help.

CHAPTER 9

Vitamin C Conquers Viral Diseases

"EARLY BUT suggestive evidence ... seems to support the contention of Linus Pauling, Ph.D., that **megadoses (massive doses) of vitamin C may palliate or prevent viral infections and possibly cancers as well, while not causing any side effects**," says *Medical World News* in its February 2, 1977 issue.

The evidence comes from Dr. Benjamin V. Siegel, Professor of Pathology at the University of Oregon Health Sciences Center. Dr. Siegel does not completely agree with Dr. Pauling on how this virus-killing procedure may work. He thinks that two things are involved.

First, he says vitamin C produces large doses of a protein substance called Interferon. The medical dictionary defines this as a body protein which, in the presence of a virus, prevents the virus from reproducing and can also create resistance to a variety of viruses. In other words, a cold virus or a polio virus enters the body, the interferon goes to work to prevent it from spreading and overwhelming the body's defenses. It also makes the body resistant to the virus, so that it will be able to fight off some future attack by the same virus

If this is indeed the case, **massive doses of vitamin C appear to be the single most effective medical weapon yet discovered,** since we have, up to now, no drugs to fight viruses and no way to protect from viral attacks in the future except vaccination. If, as Dr. Siegel says, **massive doses of vitamin C are also completely without any harmful side effects**, this would be the first time any virus-fighting weapon has been discovered that did not have side effects—perhaps very serious side effects.

The second operation of vitamin C in the presence of a virus is to activate certain blood cells which are formed in the lymph glands in many parts of the body. They are called lymphocytes. Their job is also to surround invading viruses or bacteria and destroy them before they have a chance to multiply and spread throughout the body, doing vast damage.

What is a virus? According to *Gould Medical Dictionary*, it is "a vast group of minute structures, in the range of 250 to 10 millimicrons, composed of a sheath of protein encasing a core of nucleic acids, capable of infecting almost all members of the animal and plant kingdoms, including bacteria, characterized by a total dependence on living cells for reproduction and lacking independent metabolism."

Leukemia is a disease of the blood forming organs, characterized chiefly by uncontrolled proliferation of the leukocytes—the "white" blood cells. Dr. Siegel infected two groups of laboratory mice with large amounts of leukemia virus. One of these groups had gotten massive doses of vitamin C for three months before the experiment began. The other had not. The mice which had been given vitamin C produced 10 per cent more interferon and developed milder leukemia than the controls. Dr. Siegel is now using smaller doses of the leukemia virus to see if the large doses of vitamin C can entirely prevent or delay the onset of leukemia.

"There is already solid evidence in the (medical) literature," says Dr. Siegel, "that macrophages—those 'angry' cells—are enhanced by interferon and that any agent that stimulates interferon might thus in turn eradicate

72

viruses of cancer cells. We've inferred that vitamin C may be that agent in this case."

He goes on to speculate that cold viruses get into the nose, their presence stimulates the production of the protective substance, interferon, which spreads to neighboring cells, producing more and more of their defensive substance, thus preventing the virus from spreading.

Dr. Siegel agrees with other aspects of Dr. Pauling's theories as to how vitamin C strengthens the body's defenses against viruses.

"The more experiments I do," Dr. Siegel says, "the more vitamin C I take. The dose I give these mice is of the order of 15 grams a day for a 150-pound man and I've gone from taking 250 milligrams to two grams a day. While I wouldn't want to make the jump to having every physician, say, cure hepatitis with vitamin C, I would say that more experiments should be done with humans with large doses."

Dr. Robert Cathcart III of Nevada is an orthopedic surgeon who, for the past five years, **has been using vitamin C in massive doses to cure viral diseases and treat many other conditions of ill health.**

Speaking at a meeting of the California Orthomolecular Medical Society in February, 1977, Dr. Cathcart described his practice involving 5,000 patients in which time not a single patient of his suffering from a viral disease had to be hospitalized. Viral pneumonia, mononucleosis, "flu," colds, hepatitis, shingles, cold sores and all children's viral diseases are some of the conditions he treats regularly with large amounts of vitamin C, taken by mouth or, in more serious cases, intravenously.

He believes that any viral disease now or in the future can be conquered by large doses of vitamin C. He does not know how or why the vitamin succeeds where everything else fails. He knows positively, he says, that if the vitamin is given in large enough doses, it detoxifies the virus, destroys the associated poisons which the disease has created and leaves the patient clinically well without side effects or

73

after effects.

There are 100-gram viral diseases and 50-gram viral diseases, and 200-gram viral diseases, says Dr. Cathcart. By this he means that it will take 100 grams of the vitamin to cure one disease, 200 grams to cure another, or possibly 50 grams to cure a third. And, of course, one must also consider biochemical individuality, since each patient is different and may require individualized dosage.

The cut-off point is determined by the appearance of diarrhea. This, he says, is your body's way of telling you, "That's enough vitamin C. Don't send down any more." Of course, diarrhea may be caused by many different things. You have to be certain that none of these is bothering you, that it's the vitamin C which has overpowered your colon's ability to deal with it.

The reason for this diarrhea (which is the only side effect Dr. Cathcart has encountered) is probably easy to explain. Almost all other animals, except human beings, make their own vitamin C in their livers. They make enormous amounts of it, especially when they are under any kind of stress. Disease is a form of stress. The vitamin C is conducted to every cell by the blood and does not go through the digestive tract.

Human beings, eating fruit and vegetables, get a certain amount of vitamin C in their food and their digestive tracts are equipped to handle this without any problems. But when massive doses are taken, the digestive tract in some individuals may rebel after a time. If it does and diarrhea results, then the dose must be reduced, says Dr. Cathcart. So long as diarrhea is not present, the large doses are beneficial and the sicker you are the more vitamin C you need.

At the time the swine flu vaccine was being given, Dr. Cathcart and his daughter did a test on themselves. They used a tongue test by which you can roughly determine the body's supply of vitamin C. This test, taken before the swine flu shots, showed that the bodies of both Dr. Cathcart and his daughter were well supplied with vitamin C. The day *after* they got the shots they used the test once again and found there was almost no vitamin C left in their bodies. A few days later the usual level of vitamin C was restored.

Dr. Cathcart thinks this shows that vaccinations create a condition in the body in which large amounts of vitamin C are required and are destroyed. His experiment does not demonstrate that one should never get a "shot" to protect him from a viral disease. It does seem to demonstrate, however, that the shot itself is a powerful form of stress and the body needs large amounts of vitamin C to overcome this stress and carry on normal activities. It seems to us that the elderly people who died after getting the swine flu shot possibly died from the attendant stress and not enough vitamin C to protect them against the stress. Generally, older folks don't have a great deal of vitamin C in their bodies to tide them over such an emergency.

How does it happen that some physicians who decide to treat patients for colds using vitamin C haven't succeeded? Well, says Dr. Cathcart, a patient may come in with a 100-gram cold and the doctor prescribes four grams a day. It's not likely to cure the cold, so the doctor will be convinced, after several such experiences, that vitamin C just doesn't cure colds. If the patient has a 4-gram cold, the doctor will succeed in curing it and this doctor will be convinced that vitamin C is indeed powerful against colds.

The vitamin doesn't necessarily work rapidly, says Dr. Cathcart. Often it takes just as long to cure a cold with vitamin C as without it. But the patient is hardly sick at all. He can easily go to work and carry on all other activities with no difficulty. He does not experience the usual side effects. And the cold does not develop into pneumonia or something else that is very serious.

What about the possible side effects of massive doses of vitamin C which opponents of this therapy have warned against? Is it possible that large amounts of vitamin C may destroy all the vitamin B12 in the body, thus producing pernicious anemia? Is it possible that the vitamin C may produce oxalate stones in bladder or kidneys? **Dr. Cathcart says he has used these massive doses for five years on 5,000 patients and has never seen a case of pernicious anemia develop, never seen a kidney or bladder stone develop.**

In serious cases of viral diseases where the patient cannot tolerate more vitamin C by mouth, Dr. Cathcart regularly administers the vitamin by intravenous drip in a special preparation designed for this kind of therapy and gives a calcium drip along with it. He has given, he says, a total of 215 grams (215,000 milligrams) a day to a very sick patient, by mouth and by intravenous drip. The patient recovered completely.

Other case histories sound almost as unbelievable as this one. They can be explained only by the fact that, as we pointed out above, the sicker you are the more vitamin C you need. Very sick patients have no difficulty in dealing with doses as high as 100 grams a day. That's 100,000 milligrams.

Dr. Cathcart has also used vitamin C against **scarlet fever and bladder infections, penicillin rash, bee stings, poison oak, hangovers, tooth extractions, injuries and urethritis.**

The inflammatory disorders are also likely to yield to large enough doses of vitamin C—things like bursitis, tendonitis and even arthritis—usually in cases of very elderly debilitated people.

Shingles is the agonizingly painful viral infection of a nerve system. Dr. Cathcart says it can easily be cured with very large doses of vitamin C. And if these large doses are continued for two weeks the infection will not return. In many cases where nothing but pain-killers are given, it does return and may last for months or years.

Dr. Cathcart says he has found that **the average person can take as much as 10 to 15 grams (10,000 to 15,000 milligrams) of vitamin C when they are well, with no threat of diarrhea.** If they have a slight cold they can take as much as 30 to 50 grams of vitamin C—that is, 30,000 to

50,000 milligrams—with no diarrhea. Patients with **infectious mononucleosis** can easily take as much as 200 grams (200,000 milligrams) daily with no problems.

Dr. Cathcart believes, he says, that these wide differences in "tolerance" indicate degrees of absorption in the bowel. Well people will absorb as much as they need for good health. If they take too much, some of the vitamin C is not absorbed and creates diarrhea. In the case of illness, the patient needs so much more of the vitamin that every bit of it is absorbed. **So the amount of vitamin C you need varies from day to day.** If you are beginning to get a cold you will be able to take far more vitamin C than you usually do. Then, too, if you are under stress you will be able to take more than when you are not under stress. No one but you can determine how much you should be taking every day. It's a challenge.

Dr. Cathcart regularly cures bladder infections with massive doses of vitamin C. He has used it successfully to treat **scarlet fever, hay fever, insect bites, etc**. He has used it for **arthritis, bursitis and tendonitis**, but you really have to "pour it on" in some cases, he says. One would think that anyone suffering from these excruciatingly painful disorders would not mind "pouring on" the vitamin C if there was a chance of relief.

Recent headlines in most newspapers and magazines have indicated that a ferocious battle is going on among leading individuals and organizations involved with science, health and medicine. The focus of the fight is Dr. Linus Pauling and his theories on vitamin C. Some prestigious scientific journals have refused to publish his articles.

The deliberate attacks began in earnest several years ago when Dr. Pauling wrote what turned out to be the most controversial book that ever set scientific tongues to wagging and tempers to flaring. He dared to state in the book, *Vitamin C and the Common Cold,* and to back up his statements with abundant evidence, that taking large amounts of vitamin C when the first symptoms of a cold appear will stop the cold or, if it develops, will shorten it and alleviate the most serious symptoms.

All the many critics of the habit of taking vitamins went wild for this man was proposing massive amounts of vitamin C—up to 10 grams a day. Most medical journals and many prominent nutrition specialists jumped on the "get Pauling" bandwagon and rushed into print with denunciations of such a ridiculous, not to say dangerous, idea and warned of terrible health consequences to anybody who followed this crazy man's advice.

But Dr. Pauling, perhaps the most creative and distinguished biochemist alive, does not take kindly to being kicked around, especially by critics who had obviously not even bothered to read his book. He fought back, answering every attack with calm repetition of the evidence he had presented in his book. The book is by now a classic and many of the critics have had to eat their words.

In a second book, *Vitamin C, the Common Cold and the Flu*, Dr. Pauling tells the full story of everything that went on around the first book, and answers all the complaints again, fully and unemotionally. Dr. Pauling gives us more information on all the tests that have been run on vitamin C and colds. He analyzes the position of the medical profession in regard to his theories on vitamin C. **He compares vitamin C to drugs in its usefulness and its lack of potential for physical harm.** He discusses swine flu and tells us, "The measures to be taken for the prevention and treatment of influenza through use of vitamin C are essentially the same as for the common cold . . . For most people the regular intake of vitamin C should not be used as an excuse for continuing to work until exhaustion sets in."

In one stunning chapter, Dr. Pauling theorizes on **the possibility of using vitamin C for many other disorders, chiefly those of viral origin:** viral pneumonia, hepatitis, polio, tuberculosis, measles, mumps, chicken pox, viral orchitis, viral meningitis, shingles, fever blisters, cold sores and canker sores.

The book is another challenge to the doubters and to Dr.

Pauling's critics. They will, no doubt, attack it as savagely as they did his first book. Never mind. For those of us who already know the benefits of vitamin C, the new book provides much new ammunition for convincing our friends and relatives. Dr. Pauling lays low the fears about vitamin C using up all the vitamin B12 you may have in your system, the fears about the possibility of kidney stones from massive doses, and all the other imagined harms that columnists and official spokesmen for this or that medical group have headlined.

Get a copy of this book for yourself, your doctor and one for the local public library if it is not already there. The book is published by W. H. Freeman Company, 660 Market Street, San Francisco, California 94104.

We think that the work of Dr. Siegel, Dr. Cathcart and Dr. Pauling is one of the most important contributions of our time to an understanding of how and why vitamin C may play an absolutely essential role in protecting us from viral and bacterial diseases. This is the most encouraging news we have had about viral diseases in a long, long time.

Don't you agree? And don't you think it's very, very wise to maintain your store of vitamin C at a high level all the time, since you are continuously encountering viruses and bacteria of differing toxicity, some not so toxic, others deadly. It is becoming increasingly evident through experiments like these that the idea of taking every day only enough vitamin C to prevent scurvy is like drinking only a few drops of fluid every day—just enough to keep from dying of thirst! How much more healthy we are when we can drink all the water we want to drink, and take all the vitamin C we need to prevent many health atrocities!

CHAPTER 10

Vitamin C
for Your
Back Troubles

BACK PAIN seems to afflict just about everybody at one time of life. Statistics collected by writers on the subject seem to show that, during any given year, 28 million Americans may stagger into their doctors' offices doubled up with pain in (usually) the lower back region. Since President Kennedy's famous rocking chair made its appearance in the White House, lower back pain has become fashionable. In almost any gathering at least some people present can boast of their sacroiliac or "slipped disc" complications.

There seem to be three main reasons for today's epidemic of back troubles. First is the structure of the human back which readily lends itself to poor alignment. We were probably meant to walk on all-fours, as other mammals do. When our early ancestors began to walk upright, the spinal column had to absorb all the extra work and accommodation. Somehow this curiously complicated string of bones and nerves had to become adjusted to carrying weights, walking on hard surfaces, bending suddenly to pick up heavy loads, sitting all day working at a desk or machine, riding all day and/or night in a jogging truck or automobile. We further complicated things by wearing shoes with heels which throw us even further off balance. And we became, over the past 40 years or so, almost sedentary. And that brings us to the second probable cause of most back troubles—**we just don't move around enough**.

Dr. James Greenwood, Jr., Professor of Neurosurgery at Baylor College of Medicine and Chief of Neurosurgery at the Methodist Hospital in Houston, Texas, says in *Executive Health*, Volume X, No. 12, that spinal discs, the joints that accompany them and the ligaments that tie the joints together have no significant blood supply of their own. They are, he says, "dependent upon motion for the introduction and distribution of nutrient fluids." In other words, if you don't move around enough, especially if you don't use your back regularly and intensively all day for all the motions that a back is capable of making, you are doing yourself grave harm. **Your back, as well as other parts of you, was meant to move vigorously.**

As we of the technological age hand more and more of our hard physical work over to machines, as we ride instead of walking, punch buttons instead of doing laundry or washing dishes, turn a faucet rather than pumping a hand pump, parts of our bodies begin to show stress from not being used enough. A protracted illness or convalescence which confines us to bed for a long time further debilitates muscles and ligaments of our backs. If, unused to heavy exercise, we bend all our energies to shovelling snow or spading up the garden, we are likely to develop one of those locked backs, unable to straighten up without unearthly pain.

A third cause of modern back troubles seems to be a plain deficiency in vitamin C. It's not that we're neglecting our ritual glass of orange juice or tomato juice at breakfast, but that, somehow, in all the stresses and environmental pangs of modern life, we seem to need far, far more vitamin C than we get in the average American diet if we want to keep our backs free from pain.

At least that's the way it seems from the experience of some very **knowledgeable physicians who use vitamin C in large doses to treat and prevent orthopedic back troubles**. M. L. Riccitelli of New Haven, Connecticut, tells us in *The Journal of the American Geriatrics Society*, Volume 20, No. 1, that, in 1964, a doctor named J. Greenwood, Jr. reported that he used high dosage therapy of vitamin C in more than 500 patients with low back pain diagnosed as lumbosacral sprain, disc injury with or without root involvement, or chronic degenerative disc lesions.

"A significant number of patients with early disc lesions were able to avoid surgery," he tells us. And many patients who stopped their vitamin C intake after they improved found they had to return to it if they wanted to continue to avoid their painful symptoms. Dr. Greenwood gave his patients 500 milligrams of vitamin C daily, in two doses, increasing it to 1,000 milligrams if there was any discomfort on exertion.

The same Dr. Greenwood, in *Executive Health*, tells us that **adequate protein in the diet is important in maintaining the integrity of all these complicated mechanisms in the spinal column.** But it occurred to him some years ago that deficiency in vitamin C might be just as important. Vitamin C is responsible, after all, for the health of all the connective tissues of the body—that is, the tissues that hold us together.

When he developed back trouble in 1957, Dr. Greenwood began to take 100 milligrams of vitamin C three times daily, increasing it to 500 milligrams three times daily which relieved his own pain. He found, surprisingly, that he could also prevent muscle soreness by taking vitamin C before he started on some vigorous camping trip or sailing voyage.

He began to use vitamin C in large doses for his patients. His patients had back pain, sciatica, neck pain and arm pain. Many of the back and leg pain patients came from urologists who were treating them for cystitis or prostatitis—inflammation of the urinary bladder or prostate gland. **He** thinks that the pain in these cases came from direct deficiency in vitamin C, since it is well known that any infections use up vitamin C rapidly. So not enough was available to safeguard the health of the back and leg muscles and ligaments. As his bladder infection patients continued to take large amounts of vitamin C for their back pains, they found that it cleared up the bladder infections as well. And now, he tells us, **many urologists are using vitamin C regularly against infections.**

Patients who got over their back problems tended to neglect their vitamin C, and many of them came back several years later with the same complaints. Once again, vitamin C came to the rescue. A friend of Dr. Greenwood's, an orthopedic surgeon, suggested that he try larger doses of the vitamin for better results.

Individual doses are something that must be worked out by the individual, says Dr. Greenwood. It is impossible to lay down any general rules for dosage that will apply to everyone. He tells the story of a patient of 62 who practices ballet one hour four times a week in a class of much younger students. She had an operation on a ruptured disc years earlier when she was taking 500 milligrams of vitamin C daily to prevent colds. Some knee and back troubles that developed in her ballet classes required 2,000 milligrams a day for relief so that she could return to the class.

Dr. Greenwood refers to Dr. Roger Williams' work on biochemical individuality and says that, in every case, one's own physical make-up should govern the amount of vitamin C needed to correct troubles with backs, legs, necks and arms. What is enough for some member of your family may not be nearly enough for you, and vice versa. Even laboratory animals, bred to be as identical in all their needs as possible show great differences—as much as 20 times—in their need for various vitamins and minerals. Human beings who come from a widely varied stock of ancestors must, perforce, have even greater variability in their needs.

Today, Dr. Greenwood says, he usually starts back pain

patients on 1,500 milligrams a day of vitamin C—500 milligrams with each meal. Some patients report stomach irritation, in which case he reduces the dosage. If it needs to be increased to alleviate the back disturbances, he does so. He says that **large doses of vitamin C should not be taken on an empty stomach**, but during or following meals. Some patients take as much as 4,000 milligrams (4 grams) daily without any stomach complaints.

Vitamin C is necessary for prevention of weakness and degeneration of spinal discs, says Dr. Greenwood. It is also needed for healing strains and injuries and to prevent or alleviate severe muscle soreness due to excessive exercise. He does not claim that vitamin C is the only treatment for strengthening the back, but he insists that it is one important item.

The other most important item, he says, is exercise—regular, daily, mild exercise for "circulation of nutrient fluids and metabolism of discs, tendons, ligaments, joints and all tissues of the body.... Adequate nutrition, including optimum vitamin C, and *daily* exercise, will eliminate most back pains, strains and disc ruptures," says Dr. Greenwood.

Back pain may have its origin in arthritis, but this condition, for which vitamin C appears to be very effective, may be only distantly related, says Dr. Roger J. Williams in *Nutrition Against Disease.*

Referring to Dr. Greenwood's research, Dr. Williams reports that it is possible that the benefit of vitamin C in this case is connected with its indispensability for the production of collagen, which is so important for all body structures and is essential to maintain the structure of intervertebral discs. When relatively large amounts of this harmless nutrient (vitamin C) are taken by mouth, the cells that produce collagen are able to appropriate it and are helped to do a better job, he adds.

"While medical education has put a damper on experiments in which the nutrition of arthritics might have been studied and manipulated in an expert fashion, there is excellent reason for thinking that if this were done, sufferers could get real rather than palliative relief," Dr. Williams says. "There is even a good possibility that individual arthritics will be able—if they are lucky and make intelligent trials—to hit upon particular nutrients or nutrient combinations which will bring benefit."

Dr. Williams states that he does not want to give the impression that the management of back pain, arthritis, gout, etc., is simple, but he does think that nutrition should be tried first.

"On the basis of reports presently available," he continues, "the items that certainly need to be considered are niacin (vitamin B3), panothenic acid, riboflavin (vitamin B2), vitamin A, vitamin B6 (pyridoxine), vitamin C, magnesium, calcium, phosphate, and other minerals. The objective is to feed *adequately* the cells that are involved in producing synovial fluid and in keeping the bones, joints and muscles in healthy condition."

CHAPTER 11

Gallstones

HAMSTERS ARE VEGETARIANS. So in their natural diets they get none of the fatty substance cholesterol, which is suspected by some scientists of being responsible for circulatory complications that may lead to heart attacks. **Cholesterol occurs only in foods of animal origin**—meat, fish, poultry, eggs and dairy products. Hamsters eat only vegetable foods.

Therefore, it is the usual practice to use these little rodents in laboratory experiments with cholesterol, for here the possible harm done by this fat might be expected to be enhanced, hence easier to observe and measure. An animal which has evolved over all past generations to eat only food that does not contain cholesterol probably has no biological mechanism for disposing of this fat healthfully.

And such is the case. Scientists can fairly easily produce high levels of cholesterol in the blood of vegetarian animals and thus study various methods of rendering this accumulation of cholesterol harmless. One harmful way in which cholesterol tends to collect is in gallstones, those accumulations of fats, bile salts and minerals (especially calcium) which are often found in the gall bladders of human beings. **Gallstones affect up to 25 per cent of people past middle-age.** Gallstones vary in size, color, number and structure, depending on the types of materials used to form them.

People with gallstones may not have any symptoms, but there can be a variety of telltale signs, such as bloating, belching and abdominal pain. "The abdominal pain is severe and knife-like, radiating from the right upper abdomen to the back," according to *Medigraph Manual*, by Dr. George E. Paley and Herbert C. Rosenthal. "It is caused by the movement of a stone into the duct carrying bile to the intestine."

A gallstone attack may follow a fatty meal, or it may have nothing to do with what the patient has eaten that day, Dr. Paley and Rosenthal continue. At its peak there is severe nausea and vomiting, and the patient may find it difficult to breathe. The upper abdominal wall is tender and tense. Medication may help stop the attack, or it may stop of its own accord. Between attacks the patient may be in excellent health, the authors said.

One way to dissolve these stones in some patients is to give them doses of a certain substance called chenideoxycholic acid, which is one of the substances naturally produced by the gall bladder. In the *New England Journal of Medicine* for November 25, 1976, a Czech biochemist, Dr. Emil Ginter, describes his experiments with hamsters in which he gave vitamin C along with this medication. He says that guinea pigs must have ample vitamin C in their bodies in order to produce all the various essential substances which the gall bladder produces. When they are on diets that do not contain enough vitamin C, this mechanism goes awry and there are gall bladder complications, including gallstones.

Dr. Ginter and his colleagues gave vitamin C to hamsters which were on a diet guaranteed to produce gallstones. Fewer stones were produced and the vitamin hastened the changeover of cholesterol into digestive juice. Giving large doses of vitamin C to guinea pigs also decreased the number of gallstones formed.

Therefore, says Dr. Ginter, giving the vitamin along with

the bile acid which has already been tested should hasten the transformation of cholesterol into digestive juices rather than allowing it to form gallstones.

His experiment with hamsters showed that this does indeed happen. **He suggests that vitamin C given in large doses to human beings might produce the same effects.** It should be taken for quite a long time, he says, since short-term tests (one or two weeks) do not give the desired results.

CHAPTER 12

Shingles

PEOPLE WHO have suffered from *herpes zoster* tell us there is no pain more agonizing or more intense. *Herpes zoster* is shingles. **It is caused by the same virus that causes chicken pox.** Usually chicken pox occurs only in children. Shingles occur most frequently in adults, usually older people, often people who are suffering from some other debilitating disease.

Shingles is an inflammation of the endings of nerves that supply sensation to the skin. It develops most commonly along the trigeminal nerve which crosses the face, or the nerves which cross the chest wall or the abdomen.

Symptoms are excruciating pain along the entire course of the nerve. This may last several weeks or months. Blisters—the size of a matchhead—like those seen in chicken pox, appear along the course of the nerve. They break and form crusts eventually. And long after these outward symptoms have disappeared, the pain, called post-herpetic pain, may persist until the exhausted victim is almost convinced there will never be a let-up.

In some cases—especially in older folks—the virus may attack eye nerves and bring very serious complications. Everything that can be done to assure good eye hygiene should be done. Doctors give cortisone drops in the eye.

It seems that the varicella virus which causes chicken pox

is the same virus that causes shingles. In people who have had chicken pox in childhood, the virus lingers in the body waiting to pounce on a nerve in an individual who is in a weakened state, perhaps because of old age, perhaps because of great stress or fatigue, perhaps because of some organic disease which has weakened the individual. Shingles is the final triumph of this devastating virus which preys on weakened individuals.

It's hard to diagnose shingles before the skin eruptions appear, for symptoms are the same as those of many other diseases. *Merck Manual* says that shingles must be distinguished from pleurisy, trigeminal neuralgia, Bell's palsy and, in children, chicken pox. According to the location of the nerve involved, the pain may resemble that of appendicitis, renal colic, gallstones or colitis.

One would suppose that anyone who has had chicken pox can get shingles later on, since the virus is presumably still inside the body. On the other hand, adults exposed to chicken pox can get shingles. And children near adults who have shingles can "catch" the virus and develop a case of chicken pox.

In the *Journal of the American Medical Association*, October 17, 1977, Albert B. Sabin, M.D., of polio vaccine fame, discusses the possibility of producing a vaccine to prevent shingles. There appear to be great hazards associated with such a job. It seems that a vaccine given to a child might produce shingles when he is an adult. The vaccine itself may cause shingles much later and researchers would have to wait perhaps 20 years to find out.

Any immunity granted by the vaccine might not be as long-lasting as the immunity granted by an actual infection, so there might be more risk of a severe case of shingles in adults.

Dr. Sabin takes up these objections and indicates that he does not believe they are important enough to discourage the development of a shingles vaccine. He also points out that the virus causing chicken pox and shingles is a DNA virus. Other human DNA viruses have been shown to cause cancer under certain conditions. So one must take into account the possibility that a vaccine could produce tumors. Dr. Sabin thinks it is unlikely. And he favors research to develop such a vaccine. This may be years in the future.

As in the case with all viral diseases, prevention is infinitely better than cure. Keeping one's body so healthy that no virus can find a weak spot to attack is the best idea. This is perhaps why older folks, worn out with work and other diseases, scarred and debilitated with the after effects of many conditions of ill health, as well as drugs used to treat them, are more susceptible to shingles than young people who, in general, have more vigor.

But, as we reported in another chapter, we have good evidence that viral diseases can be prevented and, in many cases, treated successfully with vitamin C. Dr. Robert Cathcart said recently in a speech in California before the California Orthomolecular Medical Society **that he could cure any viral disease with large enough doses of vitamin C, including shingles**. Dr. Frederick Klenner of Reidsville, North Carolina, who has been using vitamin C in large doses for more than 30 years, also uses very large amounts of vitamin C to cure shingles.

Dr. Cathcart, of Nevada, uses extremely high doses . . . as much as 30 to 60 grams of vitamin C to cure a cold, depending on the severity of the symptoms. Colds are caused by viruses. Sixty grams of vitamin C is 60,000 milligrams. Anyone taking massive doses of vitamin C should space them throughout the day and the night, if possible, so that the vitamin floods every cell of the body continually. For viral flu, Dr. Cathcart gives up to 100 grams of vitamin C daily.

He has never seen any deleterious side effects. He states flatly that the sick person can take much more vitamin C than the well person can without side effects. The only side effect he has observed in his patients is diarrhea. When diarrhea occurs, he says, this is an indication that the patient is getting too much vitamin C. Dr. Cathcart also says that a shingles infection treated with vitamin C does not return later on. Treated with simple pain killers, it may stay around for months or years.

The *Merck Manual*, not very likely to recommend vitamin therapy, mentions that **some physicians have had success treating shingles with massive doses of vitamin B12**. They give 1,000 micrograms intramuscularly, every day. Most physicians these days are willing to give their patients vitamin B12 injections if they ask for them. So, if you have shingles, there is certainly no harm in asking your doctor for a B12 shot every day.

And there is no reason not to have the shots if you are, at the same time, taking vitamin C in large doses at intervals throughout the day. They do not conflict with one another, nor would either one interfere with whatever pain-killing drug or drugs the doctor may be giving. Aspirin or aspirin with codeine are the usual drugs given for shingles. They work in some patients, not in others. In any case, keep in mind that **aspirin destroys vitamin C, so if you are taking aspirin, chances are you will need more vitamin C than otherwise**.

In general, calcium and the B vitamins are those nutrients which most effectively guard the health of the nerves. We do not know of any survey indicating that victims of shingles are short on these nutrients. But it seems that the best insurance against any nerve disorder would be the vitamin B complex— in large doses if you have slighted it all these years, along with plenty of calcium—most easily available in dairy products of all kinds—milk, cheese, yogurt—and/or supplements which are available at your health food store.

Neuritis frequently develops when vitamin B1 (thiamine) is inadequately supplied, reports Adelle Davis in *Let's Eat Right to Keep Fit*. "Like the brain cells, the nerves are particularly affected by this deficiency because they are exclusive sugar burners. Neuritis, which may take the form of trifacial neuralgia, shingles, sciatica, or lumbago, is characterized by a sliding scale varying from a dull ache to excruciating pain following the nerve channels. Such pain is thought to result first from the accumulation of acids and later from actual damage to the nerve cells. Headache and nerve irritation which brings about nausea and vomiting may likewise be caused by these acids," she says.

In another book, *Let's Get Well*, Miss Davis reports that the virus infections classified as herpes simplex, which appear as water blisters on the skin may occur on the face, hands, abdomen, genitals, lips (cold sores or fever blisters), inside the mouth, and as shingles, usually respond quickly if vitamin B6 (pyridoxine), vitamin C and pantothenic acid, another B vitamin, are taken with highly fortified milk around the clock. The recipe for this fortified milk is given on Page 413 in her book.

Elsewhere in *Let's Get Well*, Adelle Davis says, "In general, the more serious the illness, the larger should be the quantity of vitamins obtained, particularly at first, and the more frequently they should be taken. For example, at the onset of an infection, one might take 2,000 to 3,000 milligrams of vitamin C, 100 to 300 milligrams of pantothenic acid, and 10 to 30 milligrams of vitamin B6, and then take half these quantities every two or three hours thereafter. If the infection is acute, the vitamins should be given every three hours during the first night, always with fortified milk. As the symptoms subside, smaller amounts can be taken, but if a relapse occurs, the quantities should be immediately increased. When recovery is complete the antistress formula (given on Page 31 in her book) may be discontinued.

"Provided the vitamins are consistently taken with a highly fortified drink, the quantities suggested here have brought excellent results to persons suffering from such a wide variety of infections as sore throats, pancreatitis, shingles, rheumatic fever, flu, infections of the sinuses, eyes, ears, or kidneys, and any of the respiratory infections," she continues.

She adds: "The rashes that occasionally occur when vitamins are taken are apparently caused by the filler

holding the tablets together and usually disappear when a different brand is purchased. Extremely large amounts of vitamin C will sometimes cause diarrhea, indicating that more is being taken than is needed; if this tendency is noticed, the amounts should be immediately decreased. . . . "

Starting right now with a program of good diet—every mouthful counting in the nutrient score with not a single empty calorie food among them—plus vitamin and mineral supplements every day to make up for past diet indiscretions should produce such good health that you need not worry about viruses that linger around hoping to catch you in an unhealthy state.

CHAPTER 13

Peptic Ulcer

PEPTIC ULCER, which affects some 10 to 12 percent of all Americans and makes invalids of many of them, may have many causes. **These painful ulcers are also known as stomach ulcers, gastric ulcers or duodenal ulcers.** The condition is said to occur about four times more frequently in men than in women. Usually only one ulcer forms in the duodenum—the first portion of the small intestine—but there may be many ulcers if the condition affects the stomach.

The gastric juice manufactured by the stomach contains hydrochloric acid, mucus and a ferment, pepsin, which breaks down protein in the food into simpler substances, we are told by *The Book of Health*, Third Edition, by Dr. Randolph Lee Clark and Dr. Russell W. Cumley. Sometimes the mechanism for secreting gastric acids does not shut off after all the food has been consumed, and the pepsin-hydrochloric acid mixture goes to work on the digestive tract itself.

"Thus, a peptic ulcer occurs in the walls of the stomach or the duodenum which are the regions bathed by the gastric juices," the medical encyclopedia explains. "Peptic ulcers may also occur in the esophagus as a result of the backflow of juices.

"The vagus nerve (either of two cranial nerves extending

through the neck into the thorax and the upper part of the abdomen) is believed to be largely responsible for the continuous overproduction of gastric acids. It receives stimulation from the sight and odor of food, and from the emotions. The vagus nerve is sometimes overactive at night when there is no food in the stomach. The juices go directly through the pylorus (the opening between the stomach and the intestine) into the duodenum. This causes destruction of the mucous membrane of the intestine and can result in a duodenal ulcer. Also implicated are the regulatory mechanisms of the stomach wall. The antrum, or lower portion of the stomach, contains a hormone to halt the production of acid when gastric juices begin to fill the antrum. Ulcers can be produced by a malfunction of this regulatory mechanism."

How do you know if you have an ulcer? Well, there is pain in the stomach, usually soon after eating if it is a stomach ulcer. If a duodenal ulcer, the pain may begin two to three hours after eating. The pain may vary from a mild stomach upset to an excruciating burning sensation. If not treated, the ulcer may eat through the wall of the stomach or duodenum, perforating a blood vessel and causing internal bleeding.

One determined researcher, Dr. T. L. Cleave, a retired Surgeon Captain in the Royal Navy, believes that the only cause of ulcer lies in a factor "which is operating unobtrusively in many parts of the world and is almost alone responsible—interference with the natural buffering of the gastric acid by the food, through the removal of protein in the refining of carbohydrates."

Dr. Cleave has written a well-documented, skillfully argued defense of his theory in a book, *Peptic Ulcer*, published by Williams and Wilkins, the medical publishers in Baltimore, Maryland. He is referring to what our millers, bakers and sugar refineries do to cereals and sugar cane when they make white flour and processed cereals of the former and white sugar of the latter. Most of the protein is removed, Dr. Cleave says, and **the protein is essential to protect the**

lining of the stomach from attack by digestive juices.
He recommends returning to entirely unprocessed natural
foods as the only way to end all our problems with ulcers.

Some other research on ulcers, which is really rather
closely related to Dr. Cleave's, has to do with vitamin C. It
seems that **ulcer patients may be suffering from a quite
serious lack of vitamin C,** according to a series of letters
that appeared in the *British Medical Journal.* One Glasgow
physician investigated the state of 109 ulcer patients in
regard to their vitamin C condition. He found that patients
with ulcers showed "evidence of depletion of vitamin C," as
well as patients who had other complications along with
ulcer.

Some patients who had had ulcer surgery and were in good
health were found to have normal levels of the vitamin, but
others showed depletion "despite an apparently normal
dietary intake." Dr. Iain W. Dymock concludes that
patients with duodenal ulcers are short on vitamin C.
He believes the reason may have to do with absorption. Even
though they may be getting enough vitamin C at mealtime,
the condition of their digestive tract is such that they cannot
absorb the vitamin.

In addition, he says that the antacid drugs given by many
physicians to ulcer patients may have this effect—that is, to
prevent the absorption of vitamin C. He says, furthermore,
that all his patients have responded well to vitamin C
supplements and he believes that supplements of this vitamin
may be essential for people with this condition.

Medical World News, commenting on the work of two
other Scots physicians, says that **ulcer patients generally
seem to get less vitamin C in their food.** And, after they
have had surgery for their ulcers, the level of vitamin C in
their bodies does not return to normal even though they
begin to eat plenty of vitamin C-rich food.

They quote Dr. Max M. Cohen as saying that in times of
stress there is increased use of vitamin C by body tissues,
especially wounded tissues. **In surgical patients, too little**

vitamin C may mean that a wound will not heal properly, or it may even open again, after an apparent healing.

The Glasgow doctors believe that the low blood levels of vitamin C in ulcer patients are due to just plain not getting enough of the vitamin in food. But they also speculate on how large a part lack of absorption may play, since the digestive tract must contain plenty of hydrochloric acid in order to assimilate vitamin C. Ulcer patients are given drugs to shut off the flow of hydrochloric acid in their stomachs.

As with colon polyps and other problems of the digestive system, it seems that **ulcers are never seen in people who eat wholly natural food**, which has not been concentrated to contain high levels of sugar and starch, without the protein "buffers" that accompany them in natural foods. The person eating this kind of diet would almost be bound to get more vitamin C than the person eating "the average American diet," with its relatively enormous content of processed foods. So perhaps both aspects of such a diet protect one against ulcers. When you cut out the processed foods which some researchers claim are the cause of ulcers, you also increase the amount of fresh raw foods that are eaten—foods rich in natural vitamin C.

The conclusion of the Scots physicians is, according to *Medical World News*, that vitamin C is inexpensively and easily administered in the form of tablets or capsules. In emergencies, the vitamin can be injected directly into veins. **Since there are no known hazards of vitamin C therapy, overdosage is never a problem.** Vitamin C is water-soluble and thus passes out of the body at regular intervals—in urine and feces—during the day.

Smoking may aggravate ulcer formation or delay the healing of an ulcer which has already formed, *The Book of Health* reports. Smoking is known to deplete vitamin C reserves, which, according to the above statements, would further hinder the patient's recovery.

CHAPTER 14

Colon Polyps

NO ONE KNOWS just what causes polyps of the colon or how to treat them. They are a type of tumor which may be harmless, but may progress to become cancerous.

From the Medical College of Wisconsin comes word that doctors there have been using **vitamin C in large doses to treat patients with one type of colonic polyp**. The patients all had what is called *familial polyposis*—a rare inherited condition which produces many polyps.

All but one of the eight patients treated had previously undergone surgery to remove the polyps, but had had recurrences. Dr. Jerome J. DeCosse, professor and chairman of surgery at the college, headed the research team. He said that half of the children who inherit this disease will develop many polyps by the time they are teenagers. If the polyps remain untreated, victims of this disorder die before the age of 40.

If the number of polyps can be reduced, there is a good chance that cancer of the colon can be prevented. And it appears that **vitamin C is the agent which brings this improvement about**. Note that we said the vitamin is used in massive doses.

It doesn't seem likely that many physicians know as yet about Dr. DeCosse's research, nor does it seem important if they do. Vitamin C is harmless in massive doses. Some physicians regularly give it to their patients throughout their lifetimes with nothing but excellent results. There is no reason why someone threatened with trouble from intestinal polyps should not make vitamin C a regular part of every day's vitamin intake. If the doctor is providing some other treatment, ask him if there is any reason why vitamin C should not be taken at the same time.

Chances are he'll say no, "but you're wasting your money." Dr. DeCosse didn't seem to feel that he was wasting his patients' money when he treated their polyps with vitamin C. Undoubtedly, there will be a furor in the medical journals, as there was over vitamin C for treating colds. Doctors who have never tried it and researchers who are not interested in anything new that is not a drug will probably pounce on this information and try to prove that the Wisconsin people just didn't know what they were doing, or the experiment wasn't "controlled," or something of the sort. Arguments will fly back and forth.

Fortunately, we need not wait until the issue is decided. It seems to us that anyone faced with the possibility of cancer of the colon should be willing to try anything harmless that promises relief. If the problem is specifically polyps, then by all means try vitamin C—in massive doses. **Dr. DeCosse used three grams (3,000 milligrams) daily for up to 13 months.**

Meanwhile, never forget that a great deal of research shows a clear relationship between **the health of the colon and the amount of fiber in the diet**. People who live in countries where the diet is loaded with fiber—lots of fruits and vegetables, nuts, seeds and only wholegrain cereals and breads—have almost no colonic problems, but, as soon as they move to our part of the world and begin to eat our bland, over-processed foods, they begin to develop the same elimination problems we have, with all the complications that accompany them.

So put fiber into your diet. The easiest way is to get bran—plain, unprocessed bran—at your health food store

100

and eat considerable quantities of it every day. Use several tablespoons to start with, increasing the amount gradually. You can add it to wholegrain cereals, bake it into bread, put it into salads, casseroles, meat loaves and so on. If the problem is specifically polyps, then by all means get some vitamin C and give it a try.

Incidentally, the research described above appeared in the November, 1975 issue of *Surgery*. **The researchers noted that vitamin C is known to be potent against some kinds of cancers.** So clearing the colon and rectum of polyps may prevent cancer. The vitamin C was given in timed-release capsules, so that it would be present at all times in the blood.

CHAPTER 15

Vitamin C, Strokes and Parkinson's Disease

AN IMPORTANT STATEMENT on vitamin C in relation to strokes appeared in the January 31, 1976 issue of the British medical journal, *The Lancet*. In the article, Dr. Geoffrey Taylor writes about the beginning of the process that leads to **strokes**—a rupture of the lining of small blood vessels of the brain which leads to degenerative changes in those blood vessels.

"I have seen similar vascular changes under the tongues of elderly people," says Dr. Taylor, "and less striking changes in younger people which I have related to low vitamin C levels. These changes are rare in vegetarians who have a lot of vitamin C in their diets and in their blood. Over 200 years ago James Lind described 'varicose veins under the tongue' as a sign of scurvy (the vitamin C-deficiency disease)."

Dr. Taylor goes on to say that in guinea pigs as well (one of the few creatures besides human beings that do not manufacture their own vitamin C), induced scurvy produces changes like this: thinning of the walls of the small blood vessels, disappearance of a certain kind of tissue and dilation of small blood vessels with hemorrhages when they are injured.

American observers, he says, have noted that **thyroid and adrenal glands are affected by low levels of vitamin C.** The fragility of small blood vessels is increased when vitamin C is lacking and the walls of these tiny vessels become much stronger when enough vitamin C is given. **Diabetics, he says, probably need more vitamin C than non-diabetics**, since they are highly susceptible to circulatory disease.

Many old people and others who eat "institutional meals", hospital food or instant meals from dispensers have permanently low levels of vitamin C in their blood, because such meals cannot contain much of the vitamin. We know that vegetables kept warm for even a brief time on a steam table lose most of their vitamin C by the time they come to the table.

Dr. Taylor tells us, further, that **vitamin C levels are low in hospital patients**, in anybody who has just recovered from a cold, anyone who has had a heart attack, who is in shock or suffering from an infection. Deaths from heart attacks and strokes increase in number during winter when the need for vitamin C is greatest and when there is the least vitamin C in daily food.

He says he often notices small hemorrhage (black and blue marks) in the arms of people whose blood pressure has been taken. These marks occur just below the cuff of the blood pressure gage. This suggests, he says, that low levels of vitamin C, especially in people with high blood pressure, can cause similar small hemorrhages in the brain and in the muscle which surrounds the heart, resulting in stroke or heart attack.

Then, too, low levels of vitamin C may disrupt the levels of fatty substances in the blood bringing increased cholesterol in the blood and surrounding tissues. This may be one of the causes of cholesterol deposits in the process of hardening of the arteries, which is present in most circulatory disorders.

All this suggests, says Dr. Taylor, that doctors begin to reassess the significance of low levels of vitamin C which may be chronic or may just occur from time to time. These low levels may be, he says, factors in the cause and prevention of strokes which are one of the most feared of all complications of circulatory disease.

In *Food Facts and Fallacies*, Dr. Carlton Fredericks and Herbert Bailey tell the story of a Monsignor in the Catholic Church, in his late 70s, who had suffered a stroke that had left him partially paralyzed and unable to speak. His physician wanted to restore the Monsignor's health sufficiently so that he could attend the 50th anniversary of his ordination. The physician and Dr. Fredericks, as a consultant, were given three months to perform the near-miracle.

"The Monsignor attended his anniversary, and was able to make a short address," Dr. Fredericks and Bailey report. "One of the nutritional therapies we used that made this possible comprised large doses of vitamin C, the bioflavonoids and vitamin E. **Vitamin E helps the body to absorb blood clots.**"

In a later book, *Psycho-Nutrition*, Dr. Fredericks blames the 120 pounds or so of sugar eaten by Americans each year as a major cause of stroke and other debilitating illnesses. Sugar is thus supplying more than 20 per cent of the calories in many diets, he says.

"In addition to helping to incite vitamin deficiency, hypoglycemia, and diabetes, such a physiologically unhealthy amount of sugar tends, in 70 per cent of its consumers, to increase fasting levels of blood insulin, cholesterol, cortisol, uric acid and triglycerides. It increases the production of hydrochloric acid and pepsin in the stomach, raises the adhesiveness of blood platelets, and induces the body to part with chromium—a metal needed for proper metabolism of sugar.

"It is conducive to constipation and to increased stool transit time, which may be implicated in disorders of the digestive tract ranging from hiatus hernia to diverticulosis to bowel cancer," he goes on. "It causes enlargement of the liver and, to a lesser degree, of the adrenal glands, and shrinkage of the pancreas. All this translates into sugar acting as a stress on the organism, pushing the body in the direction of diabetes, coronary heart disease, stroke, gastric ulcer and atherosclerosis."

In the March, 1975 issue of *The Lancet*, two American doctors report on treating a **Parkinson's Disease** patient with a drug which is often used in these cases—levodopa.

Parkinson's Disease, also known as shaking palsy, is a nerve and muscle disorder which may bring tremor of hands, head or arms; a peculiar gait; excessive saliva or drooling; muscular rigidity; slowness of movement; difficulty in speaking; bizarre tics and other distressing symptoms.

Little is known about the cause of the disease, according to *Medigraph Manual*, by Dr. George E. Paley and Herbert C. Rosenthal. One reason may be degenerative changes in certain areas of the brain occurring in old age. Head injuries have been suspected, but evidence doesn't support this. A condition resembling *Paralysis agitans* (Parkinson's Disease) follows encephalitis and sometimes syphilitic infection of the central nervous system. It occurs most often in men in their 50s and 60s.

Patients who are confined to bed with this disorder often develop pneumonia, bladder infections, kidney stones and bed sores.

The Book of Health, Third Edition, by Dr. Randolph Lee Clark and Dr. Russell W. Cumley, reports that the disease is related to the encephalitis lethargica epidemic of 1915 to 1926. This virus disappeared in 1931. In persons infected at that time, they say, the virus is thought to have damaged or lain dormant in the part of the brain that controls muscular movements. Only one victim of this disease born since 1931 has been reported by one group of investigators.

The patient described in *The Lancet* article had shown dramatic improvement in his condition when the drug levodopa was first given. But the drug produced such nausea that he was unable to continue with the treatment. The doctor reduced the dosage. The patient's nausea continued, only a little less than before, but the initial improvement did not. The doctors decided to give vitamin C—one gram (1,000 milligrams) a day, gradually increasing to 4 grams a day. The levodopa dose was decreased.

Almost at once, the doctors say, the nausea disappeared. **Within four weeks of taking these large doses of vitamin C, the patient's symptoms were much improved.** He was able once again to move his head normally and to play the organ, something he had not been able to do for several years. Salivation also decreased, and his speech and handwriting improved considerably.

The physicians thought that the increased attention they were giving him might be responsible for the improvement. So, without telling the patient what they were doing, they substituted another pill for the vitamin C pill. All the improvement disappeared within two weeks. Excess salivation returned. Nausea returned. Coordination deteriorated. The doctors started the vitamin C pills again and once again improvement began to show within a short time.

The case of one patient is not an indication that all Parkinson patients will respond this way, say Dr. William Sacks and George M. Simpson of the Rockland State Hospital, Orangeburg, New York, but they think that more doctors should try this treatment and see if they get similar results.

There is no indication that the vitamin C was "curing" the Parkinson's Disease. But the drug which brought improvement for the disorder could be safely given if the vitamin accompanied it.

If Parkinson's Disease is indeed caused by a virus or viruses, vitamin C is certainly useful. In another chapter, we discuss how vitamin C is useful in treating a wide range of viral diseases. Vitamin C would also help the patient who develops pneumonia, infections, etc. It seems a harmless remedy to give large doses of vitamin C—along with the only drug which has proved effective in treatment of Parkinson's Disease, if your doctor approves it.

Drugs can also cause Parkinson's Disease. The medical dictionary calls this disorder "idiopathic," which means "of unknown or obscure cause." *The Merck Manual*, 12th Edition, says, in addition, "Symptoms resembling Parkinsonism may result from carbon monoxide or manganese poisoning. Patients taking phenothiazine or reserpine tranquilizers may develop symptoms typical of Parkinsonism, which usually disappear when the drug is withdrawn."

In a book on manic-depressive illness, *Moodswing*, by Ronald R. Fieve, M.D. (published by William Morrow, New York), Dr. Fieve says, of one patient he is describing, "During her first weeks on the ward she did not sleep and was in constant motion, talking too fast and annoying the staff. By Day 10 the dosage (of tranquilizers) had reduced her pyschotic behavior, but had also introduced rather unpleasant side effects, including muscular rigidity and the masklike face of mild Parkinsonism which most major tranquilizers are known to produce...."

By 1963, about 95 million prescriptions for mind-altering drugs were being written in this country. The tranquilizers alone were being regularly consumed by one adult American out of every 12. By now, these figures have skyrocketed. As we know, tranquilizers are now being given to millions of school children to keep them quiet and manageable in classrooms. The mind boggles to contemplate what legions of Parkinson's patients our doctors will have to treat in future years. If you know someone who is taking tranquilizers, why not show him this story and ask if he can't devise better ways to keep his nerves calm and avoid anxiety.

CHAPTER 16

Vitamin C, Zinc
and the
Hazards of Alcohol

Two ESSENTIAL, life-saving nutrients have now been shown to be useful in preventing some of the worst effects of heavy drinking. Two researchers at the Oklahoma City Veterans Administration Hospital injected laboratory mice with enough alcohol to kill them, or almost kill them. Some of the mice had been given large amounts of vitamin C before the injection. All of these animals survived. The rest died.

Another group of mice, injected with alcohol, was given the trace mineral zinc before the injection. Of these animals, 90 per cent survived. Of those mice which got no nutritional support, less than one-third survived.

In another experiment, rats were injected with alcohol at frequent intervals for four weeks. They became what, in human beings, is described as chronic alcoholics. An hour after each injection the alcohol was measured in their blood. In animals which had been given vitamin C before the injections, the level of alcohol was considerably lower than in those which got no vitamin. The same was true of zinc.

The researchers say, as researchers always do, that their

experiments only partially support the theory that the same might be true of human beings given enough zinc and vitamin C. Research is continuing, they say.

We say, research or no research, alcohol or no alcohol, all of us should be getting far more vitamin C than we usually get and far more zinc than we get in the average American diet from which this trace mineral and all other trace minerals have been removed almost completely, when grains are refined to make white flour and processed cereals. White sugar is another food which presents the body with enormous problems of metabolism and no vitamins or minerals to help in the complex enzyme systems involved. They have all been removed when the sugar was refined.

Alcohol is a poison. **Enough vitamin C is a protective shield against many poisons.** Now it appears that alcohol is one of these. **Zinc is used by the body in dealing with all carbohydrates.** This is why it is so essential for those with low blood sugar or diabetes. There is no zinc in any alcoholic drink, just as there is no zinc in sugar or white bread. So increasing your intake of these substances is bound to leave you deficient in zinc.

The body organ which contains more zinc than any other is the male prostate gland. How much of our modern epidemic of prostate disorders is the result of 100 years or so of large amounts of sugar, white flour and booze? All of them make immense demands on the body's supply of zinc and provide no zinc to help on this metabolic work.

A possible relationship between vitamin C and the ill effects of alcohol was found by four Scots physicians and reported in *The Lancet* for September 21, 1974. These doctors, from the Stobhill General Hospital tell us that alcoholics suffer from many nutritional deficiencies. **Subclinical scurvy associated with an inadequate intake of vitamin C is common among alcoholics.** This means a condition not serious enough to bring on full-blown symptoms of scurvy, but almost that serious.

Vitamin C works with an enzyme in the liver which is

concerned with treating alcohol safely and sending it along to be dissolved into harmless metabolites. To see if this theory is correct, the four physicians gave one gram of vitamin C daily for two weeks to a group of volunteers, then gave them alcoholic drinks. Testing the amount of vitamin C in the blood and the amount of alcohol in the blood, they found that, the more vitamin C present, the less alcohol.

Apparently the vitamin had functioned with the liver enzyme to process the alcohol, removing it from the blood. The liver enzyme, called *alcohol dehydrogenase*, is the principal body enzyme involved in disposing of alcohol, say these authors, so, therefore, it seems that the effective functioning of this enzyme is dependent on being saturated with vitamin C.

Commenting on these findings, *New Scientist* for September 26, 1974 said, **"Drinkers may therefore like to add vitamin C to their list of 'professional' remedies."**

We would point out that **the B vitamins, too, are vitally concerned with the body's use of carbohydrates**. They, too, are destroyed in milling flour and refining sugar. Alcohol in even reasonable amounts depletes the body of B vitamins to such an extent that orthomolecular physicians are discovering they can cure alcoholics simply by giving them massive doses of the B vitamins and vitamin C.

If you drink, don't drive. If you drink, do take massive doses of vitamin C and the B vitamins all the time, not just when you are drinking. Get plenty of zinc in wholegrains, nuts, seeds and other foods where it is plentiful. You may be able to avoid some of the damage the alcohol is doing. You may, who knows, find eventually that you no longer enjoy drinking, that you can easily do without the usual cocktail or that third glass of wine.

For more information about using vitamins to fight the hazards of alcoholism, write to the Huxley Institute of Biosocial Research, 1114 First Avenue, New York City 10021.

CHAPTER 17

Using Vitamin C in a Doctor's Practice

DR. FREDERICK R. KLENNER practices in Reidsville, North Carolina. His reports on vitamin therapy for almost anything are not published in the slick, expensive professional journals put out by universities and research centers. He does not report on farfetched experiments on rats which continue for three or four days.

Instead his testimony burgeons with stories of patients who crowd his office to receive massive doses of vitamins and recommendations for a healthful diet. There is no experimenting for two or three days. Dr. Klenner's patients take their vitamins for life and, he reports, they remain healthy so long as they do.

In a letter to the editor in *Medical Tribune*, Dr. Klenner says "Man, in early times, like most animals today, was capable of manufacturing ascorbic acid (vitamin C) in his liver according to his needs." He then goes on to describe just why this cannot take place in modern man since we lack the liver enzyme which, in animals, does this job. Man, says Dr. Klenner, is the victim of a mutation, a genetic fault, which occurred probably back in the Mesozoic Era "when many animals like the dinosaurs ceased to exist because they were not able to meet the ascorbic acid requirements of their bodies due to ever-increasing stress and alterations in the environment."

"Man, being one of the lesser animals in stature, at the time, found it possible to secure an adequate exogenous (outside) source of vitamin C to meet the challenge," says Dr. Klenner. "An all-providing Creator, through infinite knowledge, knowing in advance of the change that would happen to planet Earth, provided ample ascorbic acid in the many things He brought forth on the third day. Man, however, as he has done with so many things, has destroyed in large part these 'natural deposits,' making supplemental requirements necessary."

We suffer from many genetic faults, he goes on. Other enzymes missing from our bodies at birth cause some of us to be unable to use some elements in food. Special diets must be planned for such individuals. But giving plenty of vitamin C will always cure a condition of scurvy which is the disease of vitamin C deficiency. According to several researchers whom Dr. Klenner quotes, based on experiments with rats, **an adult human being would naturally produce about four grams (4,000 milligrams) of vitamin C every day, if he were able to manufacture it for his own needs.** This is true if he is not "under stress."

But the rat "under stress" produces almost four times that much, relative to its weight, so presumably the human being "under stress" would need about 16 grams (16,000 milligrams) a day to survive in good condition in spite of the stress. Says Dr. Klenner, "It would seem that my observation on several thousand 'human' patients...over the past 28 years, relative to 10 grams of daily ascorbic acid as being the lowest amount necessary for maintaining good health, is correct. There is a major difference between just existing and being in good health."

He goes on to quote Dr. W. J. McCormick, who said

several years ago that about 90 per cent of all Canada's school children were suffering from subclinical scurvy—that is, a condition bordering on the deficiency disease scurvy. Dr. Klenner finds that about 85 per cent of some 500 office patients he has treated are deficient in vitamin C.

Dr. Klenner then describes an incident of which he is understandably proud: the birth of quadruplets to one of his patients. He started these tiny two-pound babies on 50 milligrams of vitamin C within hours after their birth. The amount was increased gradually. By the time they were one year old they were getting one gram (1,000 milligrams) of vitamin C every 24 hours. The babies were cared for on a plain hospital bed with no special equipment. They are now about 30 years old—the only surviving quadruplets in southeastern U.S.A.

He says that Dr. Linus Pauling's thesis about vitamin C and colds is correct "because his recommended dose of **one gram (of vitamin C) every hour around the clock will cure any virus cold**. Hornick and Schwartz (other researchers) employing only three grams every 24 hours could expect failure. When penicillin became available for general usage the dose was 5,000 units for every four hours; 10,000 units was really laying the drug in. For the same type pathological conditions today who would give less than a million units?—and that every four to six hours. It's time to become of age."

In an issue of the *Journal of Applied Nutrition*, Dr. Klenner tells some of the following stories, all having to do with massive doses of vitamin C.

He has used vitamin C for many patients with after-effects of **severe virus infections**. In 1953, he had a patient with virus pneumonia, unconscious, with a fever of more than 106 degrees. He gave her 140 grams of vitamin C intravenously over a period of 72 hours. By that time she was almost well. He believes that stubborn after-effects of virus infections are the cause of "crib deaths" that take the lives of so many apparently healthy infants. "Physicians must recognize the

113

inherent danger of the lingering head or chest cold and appreciate the importance of early massive vitamin C therapy," says Dr. Klenner.

He goes on to say that **there is a tragic lack of vitamin C in the blood of burn patients**. He treats them by enclosing the burned parts in a heated cradle-like arrangement so that nothing touches the skin. No dressings. He uses a 3 per cent vitamin C spray over the entire area, alternated with vitamin A and D ointment over the burn. He gives massive doses of vitamin C by mouth. During long periods of massive vitamin C dosage, he also gives calcium gluconate to check any tendency to form oxalic acid, which is destructive of the vitamin.

Dr. Klenner says that we are all victims of carbon monoxide, which is one of the most harmful elements in air pollution, especially car exhausts. **For carbon monoxide poisoning he gives massive doses of vitamin C** which seems able to separate the carbon monoxide from the red blood cell which it is in the process of destroying.

All the conditions listed above are conditions of stress. Animals under stress would produce enormous amounts of vitamin C, as we have seen. Human beings cannot manufacture their own vitamin C. Does it not seem likely that much more of it during stress might protect them, too, from further damage?

Dr. Klenner has used **vitamin C in massive doses in 300 consecutive pregnancy cases.** (Pregnancy, too, is stress). He believes that failure to give this vitamin to pregnant women amounts almost to malpractice. His patients experience no anemia. Leg cramps occurred in fewer than 3 per cent and then only when the patient had run out of vitamin C. Abdominal marks (stretch marks) appear on the abdomens of his patients infrequently and then usually when the women gained too much weight and took too little exercise.

Labor was short and less painful. The perineum was "remarkably elastic even 15 years later." No patients required catheterization. No infections, no cardiac stress, even though 22 of these women had rheumatic heart disease. One patient had been told by another doctor that another pregnancy would be fatal. Under Dr. Klenner's vitamin C treatment, she had two more babies, went back to teaching school and still takes 10 grams of vitamin C daily.

Dr. Klenner treats snake bite and insect bites with injected vitamin C. He believes that all diabetics should be taking massive doses of it. Lack of the vitamin is responsible for the slow healing of a diabetic's wounds, he believes. The vitamin also helps the diabetic to make better use of insulin. And it helps the liver to deal with carbohydrates. Sixty per cent of all Dr. Klenner's diabetic patients can be controlled with only diet and vitamin C—as much as 10 grams daily. The other 40 per cent need less insulin and less oral medication if they are taking massive doses of the vitamin.

Dentists tell Dr. Klenner that **500 milligrams of vitamin C prevent shock and weakness after tooth extractions**. He once watched an operation in which the intestines were so weak and "glued together" that any effort to separate them resulted in tearing them. The surgeon mended 20 such tears, then closed the abdomen as a hopeless situation. Two grams of vitamin C were injected every hour for 48 hours, then four times a day. In one week the patient was discharged. "She has outlived her surgeon for many years," says Dr. Klenner.

He gives massive doses of vitamin C for mononucleosis. As does a famous Tulane urologist, he gives 1½ grams of vitamin C daily to prevent **bladder cancer** when it is threatening, and to prevent a recurrence. Dr. Klenner believes that vitamin C is the "anti-cancer vitamin." **Ascorbic acid will control myelocytic leukemia**, provided 25 to 30 grams are taken orally each day, he says. Why not? Many disease conditions are cured by giving 5 million to 100,000 million units of penicillin as an intravenous drip over four to six weeks. "How long must we wait," he asks, "for someone to start continuous ascorbic acid drip for two to three months giving 100 to 300 grams each day for various malignant conditions?"

Dr. Klenner treats overdoses of drugs with vitamin C. Also **tetanus,** in combination with a drug. Two cases of **trichinosis** were treated with vitamin C and a B vitamin. **Corneal injury, chicken pox and sunburn are also treated with vitamin C.** He treats **alcoholics** suffering from overdoses of antabuse. He tells of doctors who use vitamin C for treating **glaucoma, fever blisters, arthritis, shingles and poisoning from heavy metals like cadmium or lead. He reminds us that plenty of vitamin C prevents the build-up of cholesterol in the blood.** "Ten grams of vitamin C or more each day and then eat all the eggs you want," he says.

Will massive doses of vitamin C cause kidney stones? The urine of someone taking massive doses of vitamin C will be so acid that formation of stones will be impossible, he says. Furthermore, vitamin C induces urination, so there is no chance that urine will collect and remain in the bladder—one of the possible causes of bladder or kidney stones.

Dr. Klenner is not talking theoretically. He gives his patients these dosages, he reports on the results. It is hard to refute his case histories and tell him his own patients so treated are not alive and well, when he sees them frequently and knows their condition.

There seems to be no ulterior motive for him to use vitamin C as he does if it does not perform as he says. Doctors who never cure any patients usually do not stay successful for very long. Dr. Klenner is not selling vitamin C. He has no commerical reason for promoting its use.

If you want to take vitamin C in large doses, there seems to be no reason not to. If you have any unpleasant side-effect, such as diarrhea, reduce the dosage. People differ. Perhaps you need less than others to overcome or prevent whatever condition you are trying to relieve. Perhaps you need more than others. Don't expect miraculous overnight cures. Your body may have been getting along on very little vitamin C for many years. If you smoke or are exposed to cigarette smoke or certain other harmful air pollutants, the vitamin C you take is destroyed very rapidly in rendering these pollutants harmless.

Getting back to kidney stones, Dr. Abram Hoffer, a distinguished Canadian psychiatrist, says that he has gone over the medical literature very carefully, and "so far there is not a single report in the medical literature where this (kidney stones) has been established, and, in fact, many physicians have recommended that vitamin C be used to dissolve kidney stones."

In his practice, Dr. Hoffer uses large doses of vitamin C, vitamin B3 and other vitamins and minerals to treat schizophrenia and other mental disturbances. "I am sure there are at least 50 theoretical dangers (of taking too much vitamin C), but this one (kidney stones) doesn't have any data yet to confirm it . . . I have given patients as much as one gram (1,000 milligrams) of vitamin C per hour, day and night, for certain conditions. I have never seen acidosis. . . ."

CHAPTER 18

Dr. Stone's Daily Vitamin C Regime

SINCE DR. IRWIN STONE is one of the world's leading authorities on vitamin C, you might wonder how much of the vitamin he consumes each day. With his permission, we reprint here parts of his own daily methods of getting large amounts of vitamin C which, he is convinced, are essential for good health.

I have been repeatedly asked for details of the daily health regime that I have been using for many years, for fully correcting our genetic defect causing the inherited liver enzyme disease, Hypoascorbemia, which afflicts 100 per cent of our human population. This was developed over the past 40 years as a result of my research on ascorbate (vitamin C) and the genetics of scurvy (the disease of vitamin C deficiency)....

All humans suffer from a potentially fatal enzymic defect that prevents us from making ascorbate (vitamin C) from blood sugar in our liver, within our bodies. Nearly all other mammals are able to do this and they produce abundant quantities of ascorbate each day to satisfy their bodily needs and to overcome stresses...

If we compare the daily rate of mammalian production of

ascorbate with the Recommended Dietary Allowance (RDA) of only 45 milligrams a day for humans, which the orthodox Nutritionists have foisted on an unsuspecting public, we find that **they are recommending 300 to 400 times less than the normal daily mammalian production, a bare subsistence level. If the other mammals produced this low amount, it is unlikely that they would even survive.**

My regime is based on the simple fact of providing for daily human intake, the amounts of ascorbate that the mammals have found necessary to make within their bodies. They make these daily amounts, not just for survival, but to maintain good health throughout their entire lifetime. The earlier one starts on this regime, the greater will be the period of full health and freedom from disease and a longer life span. Since no human escapes this genetic defect, this megascorbic regime has to be kept up for one's entire lifetime. . . .

Ascorbic acid (vitamin C) is a sour-tasting substance that can be used in various acidic foods such as fruit juices and salads and can be used as a substitute for vinegar in preparation of cole slaw and vegetable salads. Sodium ascorbate is essentially tasteless and can be added to all other foods and drinks without changing their flavor. A level teaspoon of each (in powder form) is approximately 3,000 milligrams or three grams.

A good way to give ascorbate to children without their knowing it is to dissolve the measured quantity of sodium ascorbate in their milk. **Dr. Frederick R. Klenner recommends giving children one gram (1,000 milligrams) of ascorbate per day per year of age up to age 10 and then 10 grams per day thereafter.** A six-year-old would thus receive 6 grams of ascorbate each day (2 level teaspoons) in several spaced doses. The use of a teaspoon of sodium ascorbate dissolved in a glass of milk taken before meals has been found valuable in the relief of gastric and duodenal ulcers (See chapter 21, "Ulcers" of my book, *The Healing Factor, "Vitamin C" Against Disease*).

To start the day off I take, upon arising, about eight

ounces of fruit juice to which I add and dissolve a half teaspoon of sodium ascorbate and a half teaspoonful of ascorbic acid (about three grams of ascorbate). To end the day, I repeat this before going to bed which assures me that I will not only wake up the next morning, but wake up healthy. In between, I will take, at lunch, another glass of fruit juice similarly treated as my beverage or put a rounded half teaspoonful in my soup, sandwich, salad or whatever.

We always have a sprinkler-container of sodium ascorbate next to our salt and pepper shaker so we can further sprinkle additional sodium ascorbate on other luncheon or dinner goodies. This addition to foods cannot be detected as no change of flavor results. **In the preparation of salads or cole slaw or in putting together salad dressings, my wife never uses vinegar any more but uses only ascorbic acid to give the desired tartness.** The use of ascorbic acid keeps the vegetables and fruits firm and fresh and prevents any darkening or discoloration due to oxidation.... Ascorbate should only be added to foods immediately before serving and should not be added before or during cooking.

The ascorbate intake should be varied in accordance with the extent of daily stresses, the more stress the greater the intake to compensate for and maintain biochemical homeostasis (balance) under these stresses. This can be accomplished by taking extra amounts during the course of the day. **Under conditions of heavy stress, I may reach 30 to 40 grams a day.**

In this way I get my 10 to 20 grams of ascorbate which I normally take each day. In addition to the ascorbate, I take the following levels of vitamins and minerals each day: vitamin A (20,000 I.U.); vitamins B1, B2 and B6 (50 milligrams each); vitamin B12 (100 micrograms); vitamin E (800 I.U.); niacinamide (1,300 milligrams); pantothenic acid (100 milligrams); folic acid and biotin (400 micrograms each); calcium (375 milligrams); magnesium (150 milligrams); zinc (60 milligrams). I supplement my potassium intake by using Morton's Lite Salt, a 50/50 mixture of sodium chloride (salt) and potassium chloride, available in supermarkets at about 25 cents for an 11-ounce carton. I take no vitamin D as I believe a person living in a sunny climate like ours in California does not need any extra intake.

To avoid diarrhea when first starting this regime, it is suggested that instead of beginning on the full intake of 10 to 20 grams ascorbate right from the start, that one-half teaspoon of sodium ascorbate, three times a day dissolved in food or drink at breakfast, lunch or dinner be first used (about 4½ grams). Then gradually increase the dosage each day until the optimal level is finally obtained. **If diarrhea is encountered, it can be easily controlled by reducing the dosage.** The tendency to diarrhea usually decreases when the body becomes accustomed to these high levels of ascorbate on continued use....

(Perhaps we should mention that Dr. Stone uses a powdered form of ascorbic acid, as you can see from the above, half in the form of sodium ascorbate and half as plain ascorbic acid. His book, *The Healing Factor, "Vitamin C" Against Disease*, contains 258 pages of startling and helpful information about vitamin C and its use in massive doses against many serious disease conditions. It is also available in paperback for $1.25. Ask for it at your health food store).

CHAPTER 19

Smoker's Scurvy and How to Prevent It

ONE WOULD THINK that anybody who smokes these days must have deliberately closed his or her eyes to the frightening material that has appeared from official sources as well as in general publications, on the proven danger of cancer and circulatory disorders, as well as many other kinds of damage, from smoking. **It seems incredible that anyone concerned enough about health to enter a health food store would still be smoking.** But we regularly hear from people who describe their health problems and what they are trying to do about them, then add, "Oh, yes, I smoke about a pack a day."

Dr. Irwin Stone, world champion of vitamin C and its beneficial effects on a variety of health problems—some of them recorded in this book—has written a brilliant article on smoking in relation to vitamin C. It appears in the *Journal of Orthomolecular Psychiatry*, Volume 5, No. 1, 1976. This is the publication of that group of far-sighted and innovative professional men and women who are treating schizophrenics and other mentally ill patients with massive doses of vitamins, minerals and special diets.

Dr. Stone begins by saying that, of course, the best way to avoid all health problems brought on by smoking is not to smoke. But for those people who cannot or will not stop smoking, he produces well-documented evidence covering many years of experimentation and observation showing that large amounts of vitamin C are the best protection against harm from smoking. Those of us who do not smoke can also learn a lot from this article about maintaining better health with vitamin C.

Tobacco smoke is full of poisons. Tar and nicotine are only two. Cyanide is another; and carbon monoxide; as well as arsenic and cadmium. Enough vitamin C taken by the smoker will detoxify these and the many other poisons in smoke, thus possibly preventing or postponing the fatal damage that has destroyed so many cigarette smokers. Countless experiments have shown that vitamin C, in large enough doses, detoxifies many poisons: strychnine, ozone, sulfa drugs, nitrates, phosphorus, coal tar dyes, mercury, chromates and many industrial pollutants.

Says Dr. Stone, "The literature concerning this (detoxification) is so voluminous that adequate treatment would require much more space. . . ." He gives us a lot of references to this material—all of it from respected scientific journals. **He tells us that tobacco smoke has been suspected as a cause of bladder cancer since 1931.** The 1964 *Report of the Surgeon General* on smoking concluded that there is an association between bladder cancer and smoking.

Many researchers in the past 40 years have worked with this theory. They have found that smoking does indeed put certain cancer-causing substances into the bladder. They also showed that the formation of these substances could be entirely prevented by giving enough vitamin C. One group of scientists found that the cancer-causing substance was present in large amounts in the bladders of cancer patients, in somewhat lesser amounts in the bladders of smokers and much less in the bladders of non-smokers. They also found that giving one and a half grams (1,500 milligrams) of vitamin C every day completely prevented the formation of the cancer-causing substance.

They advise their patients to take large amounts of vitamin C to prevent the recurrence of cancer. Obviously, says Dr. Stone, "it would seem implicit from their work that if the smokers had sufficiently high levels of ascorbate (vitamin C) in their urine, the bladder cancer would not have appeared in the first place."

Think of the thousands of victims of bladder cancer who could have been saved by this simple expedient of swallowing a bit of vitamin C every day!

So much for vitamin C's power in preventing cancer. How does it happen that the smoker does not have enough vitamin C in his blood to prevent this disease? Mostly it happens because vitamin C is destroyed in the process of detoxifying poisons. And tobacco smoke is a poison. So the more you smoke, the less vitamin C you have to fortify you against the harmful effects of smoking.

When you smoke, you suffer from smoker's scurvy, meaning a chronic deficiency in this essential substance, which makes you vulnerable to many more diseases like fragile blood vessels (which could lead to stroke), a tendency to hemorrhage, fewer white blood cells to fight off infections, abnormal immunity responses and improper functioning of all those body enzyme systems in which vitamin C plays a part.

For the past 40 years, scientists have been showing, in laboratories, that **tobacco smoke depletes the body of vitamin C.** Dr. Stone presents the evidence from 17 such studies. It is impossible to refute. In test tubes, in animals, in human beings, the addition of only small amounts of tobacco smoke destroys vitamin C wholesale. Smokers consistently have lesser amounts of vitamin C in their blood than non-smokers. The longer you have smoked and the more cigarettes you smoke per day, the less vitamin C you have in your blood.

Testing on men and women, one group of scientists found that heavy smoking has the same effect on the amount of vitamin C in the blood as increasing the chronological age by some 40 years! One experimenter theorized that the decrease in vitamin C is one of the causes of early hardening of the arteries in smokers. This is the condition which heralds a lot of circulatory troubles.

In smokers the vitamin C drops in the adrenal glands (which protect you from stress), in the kidneys, the heart, the liver, the spleen and the brain. It follows that the function of all these organs is disrupted and disordered. The vitamin C doesn't just happen to be there. It is there because that organ needs the vitamin C to function. The less vitamin C that organ has to work with, the less efficiently it will work. In smokers who were also alcoholics, investigators found almost no vitamin C. The combination of the two poisons destroyed it all.

The reason for all this goes back to the original investigations by Dr. Stone which demonstrated that, millions of years ago, the ancestor of all human beings lost the ability to make vitamin C in the liver. All other animals, except man, guinea pigs and apes, can manufacture this vitamin in the liver and do manufacture large amounts.

A goat, for instance, which weighs about what an adult human weighs, produces as much as 13,300 milligrams of vitamin C every day to meet its health needs. The official recommended daily allowance for an adult human being has been set as 45 milligrams. Why? Why have not our health officials set their recommendations at levels to approximate those of animals which make their own vitamin C?

The reason is that official medicine has been brainwashed into believing that the only recognizable symptom of vitamin C deficiency is scurvy—the terrible disease which wiped out millions of human beings over past centuries. Scurvy is the last step before death from vitamin C deficiency, says Dr. Stone. In no way should we decide that just enough vitamin C to keep us from dying of scurvy is all we need. It seems reasonable, does it not, that we need approximately the same amount of vitamin C other animals need for ordinary good health. As we have seen, one animal, the goat, makes for itself almost 14,000 milligrams more vitamin C than our official estimate specifies. Subclinical scurvy in human beings is the result.

Then, too, goats and horses, dogs and cats, whose livers are all busily manufacturing immense amounts of vitamin C, don't smoke and don't drink or expose themselves to the thousand and one other poisons to which most of us are exposed every day. So for this reason as well, it would seem advisable to get far, far more of this essential substance than animals seem to need for good health.

Dr. Stone believes, as do most of the physicians and psychiatrists who are treating patients with what is called orthomolecular medicine, that we should all be getting far more vitamin C than we get. The more exposure we have to poisons, the more vitamin C we should get.

Smokers who cannot or will not stop smoking should at least protect their health with large amounts of vitamin C. If they also drink, the requirement is even more urgent. If they work at a job where they are exposed to air pollutants, if they drive to work in horrendous traffic jams, if they breathe the tobacco smoke of others all day long, if they are taking dangerous drugs of any kind, it's fairly certain their vitamin C stores may be depleted by the time they get to work in the morning.

How much vitamin C should one take? Dr. Stone believes that the average human being who is not under stress needs as much as 5 to 20 grams of vitamin C daily. That is, 5,000 to 20,000 milligrams. A smoker, he says, should take three to five grams more than that for every pack of cigarettes he or she smokes. That's how terrible the danger from smoking is and that's how easy it is to give yourself at least some small protection against this poison.

The Journal of the American Medical Association for April 28, 1969 told of experiments in Canada which link smoking to a lack of vitamin C. The research was done by Dr. Omer Pelletier, who conducted his experiments with the assistance of the Canadian Food and Drug Directorate. By keeping his subjects on identical diets and giving them measured doses of vitamin C over a period of about three weeks, Dr. Pelletier found that:

1). Smokers have lower vitamin C levels than non-smokers.

2). It does not seem to matter how many cigarettes are smoked per day or how long the individual has been smoking, the vitamin level remains the same. Three volunteers who had stopped smoking three or six months earlier had the same general blood levels of vitamin C as non-smokers, so their bodies had apparently repaired whatever mechanism it is that deals with vitamin C and cigarette smoke.

3). There was no difference between sexes. Women in both groups had the same blood levels of the vitamin as the men.

4). The test doses of vitamin C which were given at 8:30 in the morning were retained better than those given at 4:30 in the afternoon. This seems to indicate that one benefits more from vitamins if they are taken in the morning, perhaps at breakfast.

5). Although earlier experiments seemed to show that vitamin C is destroyed in the body of smokers (as it is in a test tube filled with smoke), so that smokers always need more than non-smokers, Dr. Pelletier believes that his experiments show that vitamin C is just not used properly in the body of the smoker.

In 1975, Dr. Pelletier presented further evidence at the second conference on vitamin C, sponsored by the New York Academy of Sciences. The study evolved from the Canadian Nutrition Survey, which analyzed smokers and non-smokers ranging in ages from 20 to 64. The 2-year study involved 812 male non-smokers, 1,243 male smokers, 1,526 female non-smokers and 1,091 female smokers. Some of the results:

1). For those who smoke 20 or more cigarettes a day,

there is a 40 per cent reduction in vitamin C levels in the blood.

2). When smokers and non-smokers of the same age, sex and vitamin C intakes were compared, the median vitamin C levels of smokers were 30 per cent lower than the non-smokers.

3). For men aged 40 to 64, the vitamin C levels were some 50 per cent lower than the levels of women the same age who did not smoke.

"Most of the tissues damaged by smoking tend to repair themselves when smoking is stopped," according to Dr. Harold S. Diehl of the American Cancer Society. "Cough disappears in a few weeks and shortness of breath is relieved, but more slowly. Frequently considered pre-cancerous, abnormal cells in the lining of the bronchial tubes also decrease when smoking is stopped," he adds.

Dr. W. J. McCormick, a Canadian physician, reports that **the cigarette smoke inhaled from one cigarette neutralizes about 25 milligrams of vitamin C**. So the second cigarette of the day would just about rob us of our quota of vitamin C for the day, which is 45 milligrams, according to the National Academy of Sciences.

Writing in the October, 1954 issue of *Archives of Pediatrics*, Dr. McCormick says that he has tested the vitamin C levels of close to 6,000 patients and has never yet found a smoker with normal levels of the vitamin.

In the March 9, 1963 issue of *The Lancet*, three scientists describe their experiment with smokers and vitamin C. They say that they have confirmed the fact that vitamin C is destroyed in a test tube when tobacco smoke comes in contact with it. They tested an equivalent amount of air and the smoke from burning cigarette papers and found that neither of these destroys vitamin C. So it must be the nicotine in the tobacco.

Then they tested the blood levels of vitamin C in volunteers who smoked one cigarette every half hour, and in volunteers who smoked 19 to 25 cigarettes within six hours.

They could find no evidence of vitamin C destroyed, they say. But when they tested the vitamin C level in the blood of long-term smokers and compared it to that of non-smokers, they found that the levels were considerably lower in the blood of those who had smoked for some time.

"There was no evidence ... that the difference in blood-vitamin levels was due to a larger intake of ascorbic acid among the non-smokers," they said.

In other words, non-smokers were not getting more vitamin C in their food than the smokers. They were simply getting the benefit of the vitamin C they did eat. But the smokers—eating the same amount of vitamin C—were losing so much of it, due to the smoking, that they consistently showed lower blood levels of the vitamin than the non-smokers.

Smoking is not the only thing to destroy vitamin C. Drugs containing mercury, procaine, gold or lead destroy vitamin C, as do antihistamines and sulfa drugs.

CHAPTER 20

Vitamin C and Fluoridation

GETTING ENOUGH VITAMIN C appears to protect against the dangerous effects of too much fluoride. It also appears to help incorporate fluoride into teeth in non-destructive amounts.

These contradictory aspects of the water fluoridation controversy are brought out by John A. Yiamouyiannis, Ph.D., who has become very active in the fight against fluoridation. In a well-documented article (21 references), Dr. Yiamouyiannis tells us that mother's milk contains as little as 0.01 to 0.05 parts per million of fluoride—almost none. However, commercial baby food contains as much as 1 to 2 parts per million. This seems to indicate that these products are manufactured in areas where the water is fluoridated. So infants who are fed commercial baby food start life with an accumulation of fluoride much higher than that of breast-fed infants.

As long ago as 1930, scientists discovered that **fluoride in food and water seems to cause scurvy-like symptoms.** Sure enough, in such cases, they found low levels of vitamin C in the blood. Scurvy is the vitamin C deficiency disease.

In 1954, in an area where drinking water contained only

0.34 to 0.8 parts per million of fluoride (much less than the recommended amount for fluoridated water) almost one-fourth of the children drinking such water had mottled teeth, the earliest symptom of getting too much fluoride. The vitamin C content of the blood of most of the children was extremely low. Giving them vitamin C improved their condition.

Guinea pigs, as we know, are one of the few animals, aside from human beings, which do not manufacture their own vitamin C but must get it in food. In 1964-65 the death-rate of guinea pig populations in Australia had reached epidemic proportions, according to Dr. Yiamouyiannis. He found the story in *Nature*, the prestigious British science journal, volume 211, page 429, 1966.

Experts decided that the deaths were caused by slightly higher levels of fluoride in feed pellets. The small animals were suffering from scurvy-like symptoms, or sub-acute vitamin C deficiency. But the animals died of fluorosis or too much fluoride. The rats and mice in Australian laboratories, which were eating the same feed pellets, had no health problems. They make their own vitamin C and, like other animals, they are able to increase their vitamin C store when they are under stress or exposed to some outside influence which depletes their bodies of vitamin C. In this case—fluoride.

One might ask why, in tests on fluoride done by the United States Public Health Service, scientists do not run into similar difficulties. The reason is that our scientists do not use guinea pigs in their tests. They use rats and mice which would not have the guinea pigs' problems with fluoride and vitamin C depletion.

Dr. Yiamouyiannis tells us that articles which have appeared in our country and the Soviet Union have shown that **vitamin C can retard the development of fluorosis—the symptom of too much fluoride**. The blood of guinea pigs given fluoride had altered levels of calcium, phosphorus and sugar. Giving them vitamin C normalized all

**Preliminary Study Indicates Cancer Death Rate
Highest in Fluoridated Cities**

City	Date Fluoridated	Water	Cancer Death Rate of White Males
1. Baltimore	1952	Fluoridated	34% higher than national rate
2. Philadelphia	1954	Fluoridated	27% higher
3. New York	1965	Fluoridated	24% higher
4. Cleveland	1956	Fluoridated	22% higher
5. Detroit	1967	Fluoridated	20% higher
6. Chicago	1956	Fluoridated	18% higher
7. Houston		Non-Fluoridated	8% higher
8. Los Angeles		Non-Fluoridated	% average

these levels as well as the amounts of minerals deposited in teeth, bones and liver.

In other experiments with guinea pigs, scientists have found that adding fluoride to the diet does not make the teeth any more resistant to decay than adding vitamin C to the diet. In areas where there is little fluoride in the drinking water, giving vitamin C as a supplement leads to the deposit of as much fluoride in the teeth as is deposited in areas where water is fluoridated.

Dr. Yiamouyiannis concludes that **fluoridating water supplies is not the answer to tooth decay**. If there is not enough vitamin C in diets and diet supplements, fluoridation will lead to depletion of whatever vitamin C there is, as well as fluorosis of the teeth and abnormal levels of fluoride in blood and tissues. For a copy of the complete paper by Dr. Yiamouyiannis, send to the National Health Federation, Box 688, Monrovia, California 91016. And get plenty of vitamin C, whether your community water is fluoridated or not. Fluoride is an everpresent pollutant of food, air and water. And, as the chart shows, fluoridation is related to cancer deaths in some cities which have fluoridated water.

CHAPTER 21

Vitamin B12 and Vitamin C Are Not Antagonists

SEVERAL YEARS AGO a nutrition scientist, Dr. Victor Herbert, published a paper in the *Journal of the American Medical Association* announcing that anyone taking vitamin C at mealtime was likely to be short on vitamin B12, since, he says, vitamin C has a destructive action on the B vitamin. The implication is that the more vitamin C you take the less vitamin B12 you are going to have in your blood.

Vitamin B12 is essential to good health. It is present in any appreciable amount only in foods of animal origin— like meat, eggs, milk and, mostly, liver. People who don't eat much of such foods risk a vitamin B12-shortage in any case. This can eventually lead to pernicious anemia, a disease so serious that it was usually fatal before doctors found out that it was caused by a simple lack of a vitamin.

So, understandably, a great many people became upset by the information on vitamin B12 and vitamin C, which was picked up by newspapers across the country. It seems obvious to us that the many people who have been taking massive doses of vitamin C for many years are not perishing from pernicious anemia. And those of us who came later to a recognition of the value of large amounts of vitamin C are not experiencing symptoms of vitamin B12 deficiency.

In addition, a number of physicians, working with patients in carefully controlled conditions in hospitals **reported that they could find no evidence of vitamin B12 deficiency in their patients**—in this case paraplegics in whom the doctors were preventing bladder infections with high levels of vitamin C.

Now we have a report from Fordham Hospital and Hoffman-LaRoche in which a carefully controlled laboratory test was done to test the stability of vitamin B12 in the presence of large amounts of vitamin C. The four researchers reported on their experiment in *The American Journal of Clinical Nutrition* for June, 1976.

They describe in detail the methods they used, so that any other scientist can use these same methods and check their results. They tested the vitamin B12 content of a meal with relatively high content of vitamin B12 and a meal with not nearly so much of the B vitamin. They added vitamin C up to half a gram (500 milligrams). **They tell us that they could detect no destruction of vitamin B12 by the vitamin C**.

The doctors point out that vitamin B12 is very stable in foods since it is bound closely to a protein in the food—so closely that "a prolonged chemical attack" could be withstood and the vitamin B12 would not be separated out and destroyed. **So vitamin C simply cannot get to the B vitamin and destroy it.**

They believe that the results gotten by the earlier scientists who reported destruction of vitamin B12 were brought about by the use of inadequate methods of extracting the B vitamin from the food being tested. By using, in the present experiment, standardized and official methods, they discovered that no appreciable vitamin B12 had been destroyed by the vitamin C.

We think you can feel perfectly confident that this test was done in good faith. It can easily be repeated to confirm it.

If you are still doubtful about the possibility of losing some vitamin B12, why not pop a vitamin B12 tablet into your mouth every few days? Or buy an all-in-one supplement which contains vitamin B12. The amount in food is so very little that almost any level of vitamin B12 in a supplement is enormous by comparison. And there is no chance of an overdose. Vitamin B12, like all B vitamins, and vitamin C, is water-soluble.

After Dr. Herbert published his claim, Dr. Jean Mayer, the syndicate columnist who is now president of Tufts University, published a column repeating Dr. Herbert's claim that vitamin C destroys vitamin B12. We wrote to Dr. Mayer asking how this could be, since both are contained in liver. He did not answer.

In the April 21, 1975 issue of *The Journal of the American Medical Association*, five physicians from the Veterans Administration Hospital of the St. Louis University Group Hospitals wrote describing the condition of paraplegics in their spinal cord injury service. Paraplegics have special problems with urinary infections. Urinary infections can be troublesome and, in some cases, fatal. If they are not prevented in some way, it may be necessary to take various antibiotics for long periods of time, which can have side effects on other aspects of health.

So, say the St. Louis specialists, "As a routine procedure, all of the spinal cord injury patients on our service receive doses of (vitamin C) of more than 4 grams a day (4,000 milligrams) to enhance urinary acidity." The healthy urine is acid in character, rather than alkaline. This acidity helps to control bacteria.

In the St. Louis hospital, 10 patients aged 17 to 69 had been getting 4,000 milligrams of vitamin C daily for 11 months. All of them were on unrestricted diets and they got the vitamin in four doses during the day. This is considered the best way to take large doses of vitamin C, for the body excretes whatever excess is not needed about every four hours. So, to keep cells suffused with vitamin C constantly, it

135

is best to take the vitamin every four hours or so—say, with every meal and again at bedtime.

When the St. Louis doctors read Dr. Herbert's warnings about vitamin B12, they gave their paraplegic patients tests for vitamin B12. They found in all cases that the levels of this B vitamin were high in their blood and in three cases were very high.

Dr. Herbert was asked by the *JAMA* to reply to this letter. He said in reply that it's possible the St. Louis assay for vitamin B12 could be in error and giving results that are too high. Are you sure, he asked, that these patients don't have something also the matter with them which might cause the levels of vitamin B12 to go up in their blood although other parts of their bodies were not getting enough of it to prevent anemia? This seems to us like childish quibbling. Obviously patients under the constant daily supervision of skilled experts are not going to pine away from pernicious anemia without somebody noticing it.

Furthermore, Dr. Herbert said that he never said that everybody getting lots of vitamin C is going to develop pernicious anemia from the lack of B12. "It is quite possible that a group of patients could be taking 4 grams of ascorbic acid daily without developing vitamin B12 deficiency... moderate amounts of iron in the diet reduce the damaging effect of ascorbic acid on vitamin B12 and taking ascorbic acid between meals would be less damaging than taking it with meals." And, of course, he goes on, if anybody is taking vitamin B12 supplements then he would most likely *not* suffer from a deficiency in this vitamin if he's also taking vitamin C.

So much for the sensational headlines. Too bad everybody who read them can't also read what almost boils down to a retraction on the part of Dr. Herbert. If any of our readers are still worried about becoming anemic from taking too much vitamin C, just be sure you eat liver frequently (it has lots of vitamin B12) or take desiccated liver or take a vitamin B12 supplement.

CHAPTER 22

Is Vitamin C
an Enzyme?

DISEASES CAUSED by harmful mutations are much in the news these days. Foundations collect money for hemophiliacs and for victims of phenylketonuria, and other diseases caused by harmful mutations. Mutations are disorders of the body enzyme systems. They create disease. They can be caused by radiation, by chemicals or other kinds of injury to cells. In every case, the disease is well known to be the result of absence of a certain part of an enzyme system. Sometimes, as in the case of hemophilia, the bleeding disease, no successful drug or dietary treatment is known. Blood transfusions must be given to replace the blood lost by hemorrhaging. In the case of phenylketonuria, the disease can be controlled by a carefully regulated diet in which a certain amino acid or form of protein is omitted from the diet.

What would you say if we told you that the most prevalent disease caused by a mutation afflicts *all* human beings and one or two other animals? What would you say if we told you that this disease has inflicted untold agony and caused hundreds of millions of deaths over past centuries because no one understood the cause of the disease produced by the mutation?

And what would you say if we told you that this disease—
which we have alluded to several times in this book—which
has afflicted all human beings for perhaps 60 million years is
easily controlled by a simple dietary treatment—something
we call a vitamin?

Dr. Irwin Stone, in *New Dynamics of Preventive Medicine*,
Volume 2, 1974, presents just such a theory. The vitamin is
ascorbic acid or vitamin C. The genetically produced disease,
inherited by all human beings, Dr. Stone calls hypoascorbemia, which means in plain language, "not enough vitamin
C." In a professional lifetime devoted to study of vitamin C,
Dr. Stone has turned up some fascinating facts which confirm
his theory.

Long ago, perhaps 16 million years ago, something
happened to our ancient ancestors which made it impossible
for them to manufacture a certain substance which almost all
other animals and birds make in their livers—a liver enzyme
biologists would call it. The enzyme which we know as
vitamin C or ascorbic acid is produced in a process which uses
five other enzymes in their livers. Human beings lack enzyme
No. 4, which goes by the name of *L-gulonolactone oxidase*.
Since the liver enzyme ascorbic acid cannot be produced
without all five other enzymes, we human beings cannot
make vitamin C in our livers as other beings do.

This apparently harmful mutation occurred way back in
time. There was no science, no medicine, no way for early
human beings to deal with such a predicament, so why didn't
we all just perish, as hemophiliacs perished in the days before
blood transfusions? We didn't because this enzyme, which is
essential for life but which we are unable to make for
ourselves, is also present in fruits and other fresh growing
things which surrounded our early ancestors in the tropical
areas where they lived.

But many years later, when our ancestors had moved into
more northern areas, says Dr. Stone, "Annually recurring
epidemics of scurvy occurred in the human population in the
late winter and early spring. As you know, scurvy is the

disease of vitamin C deficiency. Each year, this scorbutic population, in which resistance to disease was so lowered, fell easy prey to the ever present viral and bacterial invaders. It is a miracle of human stamina that this defective gene did not sound the death knell for *Homo sapiens*, but survive they did at the terrible price of high infant mortality, constant sickness and early death.

"If it wasn't for this defective gene and the scurvy it causes, the ecologic crisis due to overpopulation would have occurred centuries ago. The ferocity of the great epidemics of the Middle Ages, such as the Black Death of the 14th century which killed one-third of the population in a few weeks, was the result of an infection whipping through a severely scorbutic population lacking the slightest resistance to combat the disease.

"It is of interest to note that London suffered most violently between February and May, 1349, at a time when the deprivation of ascorbate was most severe after a long scorbutic winter. Apparently we did not learn much about scurvy in the following six centuries because the high morbidity of the great pandemic of influenza of 1918 was a repetition of the same centuries-old story," Dr. Stone explains.

There were no antibiotics to kill germs. There was no knowledge of the fact that the entire population was more or less afflicted with scurvy. When, finally, in modern scientific laboratories, vitamin C was identified as the missing link in scurvy, nutrition experts decided that this substance which occurs in citrus fruits, strawberries, cabbage and other fresh foods, would prevent scurvy. A little later they decided that the amount of vitamin C that will prevent scurvy is all we need. "Scurvy has thus been regarded as a simple dietary disturbance rather than the potentially fatal genetic liver-enzyme disease it is," says Dr. Stone.

If human beings could actually produce vitamin C in their livers, as other animals do, how much would they produce? Presumably as much as other animals do, according to size, says Dr. Stone. He tells us, with references for every statement, that rats produce up to 5,000 milligrams of vitamin C per day if they are living contentedly without stress. If they are subjected to stress, their livers produce as much as 15,200 milligrams of vitamin C.

As we quoted Dr. Stone in another chapter, the goat, which weighs about the same as a human being, produces about 13,000 milligrams of vitamin C a day. The Recommended Dietary Allowance for adult human beings deemed adequate by the National Academy of Sciences is 45 milligrams a day. Says Dr. Stone, "There is a 220-fold discrepancy between what Nature provides for the good health of a goat and what this agency prescribes for man. This same National Academy of Sciences suggests 55 times more ascorbic acid in their diets for maintaining laboratory monkeys in good health throughout their lifetime than they think necessary for man." (At the time Dr. Stone made this remark, the Recommended Dietary Allowance for vitamin C was 60 milligrams a day).

Therefore, if we gage our need for vitamin C according to that of other animals, we need something slightly under 4,000 milligrams daily. Says Dr. Stone, "For thousands of centuries, man, as we know him, has been completely dependent upon his foods to supply him with ascorbate needed for his survival. In the best of times, he eked out miserable subsistence levels of a few milligrams a day from this source. When he wasn't suffering from the effects of frank clinical scurvy, he was condemned to a lifetime of chronic subclinical scurvy. Until about 40 years ago we couldn't do much about this because we were limited to the scant natural sources of ascorbate (fruits and vegetables). With the discovery and synthesis of ascorbic acid in the early 1930's and later advances in technology, we had a solution to this 60 million year old problem.

"One would think such a long-awaited solution would have been heralded as the greatest event in human history," Dr. Stone continues. "Far from this, it took another three decades just to merely recognize the problem. Even with the problem recognized, the great bulk of medical and nutritional professionals still refuse to accept it and instead are arguing for retaining the old daily subsistence levels. . . . This is why chronic subclinical scurvy is our most widespread disease."

Dr. Stone goes on to describe how **vitamin C is used by the white blood corpuscles to fight infections**. If there is not enough vitamin C the infection wins out. Vitamin C is necessary for the body to manufacture collagen, the protein "glue" that holds us together, "the ground substance of the organs, the ligaments, the walls of the blood vessels, which lends strength to bones and scar tissue in healing of wounds. . . . This could be the basis for the high incidence and morbidity of the collagen diseases among our population as well as heart and vascular diseases," says Dr. Stone. Collagen diseases include arthritis and rheumatism.

He pleads for long-term tests on large groups of people to demonstrate the beneficial effects of large doses of vitamin C. It seems doubtful that any official group will listen to him. Nutrition "experts" have ingrained in their heads the idea that vitamin C is merely a vitamin like other vitamins. They make no attempt to explain why human beings, almost alone among animals, do not make their own vitamin C. They have done little research on how and why other animals make their vitamin C. And, most important of all, they apparently do not even know that when other animals are under stress (fear, exhaustion, cold, heat, illness, etc.) they manufacture and use far more vitamin C than when they are not under stress.

When the explorer Jacques Cartier spent the winter in Canada in 1535, according to *The Book of Health*, Third Edition, it is said that his men were saved from scurvy because the Indians showed them how to make a curative brew from the growing tips of branches of the spruce and other trees.

"About this same time," the encyclopedia continues, "the Dutch Boudewijn Ronsse described the disease and indicated that oranges were curative. An outbreak of scurvy occurred

141

among the Pilgrims at Plymouth. The British naval surgeon, James Lind, caused the adoption of lime juice as a scurvy preventive by the British navy in 1795; from this custom arose the title 'limey' for British sailors."

The familiar symptoms of scurvy include swollen and inflamed, spongy gums. Vitamin C is a necessary component of the tissues of the gums which hold the teeth in place; in a deficiency, the teeth become loose and may be lost, *The Book of Health* reports. In children who lack vitamin C, the bones may be malformed. The disease is especially severe in infants, in whom there is likely to be fever, diarrhea, loss of weight and vomiting. In severe deficiencies, the book says, there may be considerable loss of blood from intestinal hemorrhages. The symptoms usually rapidly disappear when the patient gets vitamin C.

The press and general distribution magazines often report that too much vitamin C will give you **kidney stones. It's an old saw that needs debunking.** Dr. Irwin Stone quotes Dr. William McCormick of Canada who, long ago, showed in a hospital ward that people suffering from kidney stones recovered almost miraculously when they were given large doses of vitamin C. The cloudy urine which indicated that phosphates were coming out of solution—speedily returned to a bright, clear, healthy urine. Says Dr. Stone, "The ascorbate that is removed by the kidney and excreted into the urine should not be considered as 'wasted.' High levels of ascorbate in the urine bathe the tissues of the whole genitourinary tract with a bacteriostatic, antiviral, detoxicating and healing solution which tends to prevent infection and aids in the healing of any tissue injuries. It also maintains a urinary pH at a point where crystallization of calcium phosphate is inhibited and such urinary calculi (stones) avoided."

Writing in the Foreword of *Vitamin C, the Powerhouse Vitamin, Conquers More Than Just Colds*, by Ruth Adams and Frank Murray, Dr. Frederick R. Klenner says that the oxalic acid-kidney stone scare is another infamous chapter in the attacks on vitamin C.

"This big hoax, published in the general press and ladies' journals, as well as other monotonously repeated nonsense such as diarrhea on taking high daily doses of vitamin C, has been utilized for the propagation of little else than medical and news sensationalism. Manufacturers of antibiotics and various cold preparations would like people to believe such foolishness.

"After 28 years of research with really massive doses of ascorbic acid, **I can state very emphatically that you will not develop a kidney stone by taking 10 or more grams of ascorbic acid each day**," Dr. Klenner continues.

"It is physiologically impossible for such a condition to develop. Kelli and Zilva reported that nutritional experiments showed that dehydroascorbic acid is protected *in vivo* (in the body) from rapid transformation to the antiscorbutically impotent diketogulonic acid from which oxalic acid is derived. The only way oxalic acid can be produced is through splitting of the lactone ring."

Dr. Klenner adds that this happens above pH-5. The reaction of urine when 10 grams of vitamin C are taken daily is pH-6. Oxalic acid precipitates out of solution only from a neutral or alkaline solution—that is, pH-7 to pH-10, he goes on. According to Meakins, stasis and a concentrated urine appear to be the chief physiological factors. With 10 grams or more of vitamin C each day, you have an excellent diuretic. The ascorbic acid-kidney stone story is a myth, says Dr. Klenner.

If Dr. Irwin Stone's theory sounds sensible to you, if you agree with him that we and all our ancestors have been suffering from an inherited genetic defect—the inability to create an essential liver enzyme (ascorbic acid)—then doesn't it seem wise to do as Dr. Stone and Dr. Linus Pauling do—take large doses of vitamin C daily to see if it doesn't prove beneficial? Keep your vitamin C in the refrigerator, after you break the seal. This is best for all vitamin and mineral products.

CHAPTER 23

How Long Can You Store Vitamin C?

SEVERAL YEARS AGO an enterprising scientist, fired with ambition to discourage the taking of vitamins (for some obscure reason of his own), announced to the world that it is futile to take vitamin C that has been stored for any length of time. Not only does it disintegrate so that it is no longer vitamin C, but it also disintegrates into something that may be harmful!

Well, fainthearted newcomers to the field of vitamins panicked—some of them at any rate—and probably stopped taking vitamin C in spite of any advantages they had noticed while taking it.

In November, 1975, a major vitamin C manufacturer announced that they have "conclusive scientific evidence that **vitamin C tablets are both stable and safe even after prolonged storage.**" Hoffman-LaRoche stored vitamin C tablets "under normal household conditions" of storage and found that they are stable for more than five years.

They also found that whatever breakdown products occurred represent so small a percentage of the total that they do not pose any dietary or metabolic hazards. They also said that testing methods have been available for years, in reference to the earlier statements by the complaining scientist that there was just no way to analyze tablets for their vitamin C content.

The Hoffman-LaRoche study was presented by Dr. S.H. Rubin at a meeting of the Academy of Pharmaceutical Sciences. Dr. Rubin is head of applied research at the drug company and also teaches nutrition at New York Medical College.

Dr. I.J. Wilt, formerly of the University of the Pacific in California, had said earlier that **one of the breakdown products of vitamin C, when it is stored, is oxalic acid** which might accelerate the formation of kidney stones. He had not measured the amount of oxalic acid in the stored vitamin C, but just hazarded a guess that dangerous amounts might be there. The Hoffman-LaRoche scientists said they had found only negligible amounts of this breakdown product, especially compared to the amount one normally gets at meals.

"It is obvious," they said, "that the ingestion of even a number of aged tablets daily will cause practically no increase in the intake of oxalic acid. And, they continued, the amounts of filler material are extremely small in the vitamin C tablets. These might be lactose (milk sugar) and/or an extremely small amount of sodium, neither of which compares to the amount of lactose or sodium in the average diet.

This is not the first time oxalic acid has been mentioned in regard to large doses of vitamin C. We have discussed this in another chapter. Other researchers have hinted that anyone taking vitamin C is surely going to develop kidney stones because vitamin C breaks down into oxalic acid in the body. True, they have never discovered kidney stones in anybody taking vitamin C. And some physicians in this country give it to all their patients, and have been doing so for many years. Certainly if anyone had developed kidney stones from taking

145

vitamin C it would have been reported long ago in the medical literature.

Dr. Irwin Stone discusses the subject of kidney and bladder stone in his fine book—*The Healing Factor—Vitamin C Against Disease*. He tells us of a Canadian physician's research which appears to show that stone formation (whether of kidneys, bladder, gallbladder or salivary glands) arises from *a lack of vitamin C—not from too much.*

Dr. W. J. McCormick of Canada, a pioneer in vitamin C treatment for many disorders, said, "As soon as corrective administration of the vitamin effects a normal ascorbic acid level, the crystalline and organic sediment disappears like magic from the urine. I have found that this change can usually be brought about in a matter of hours by large doses of the vitamin—500 to 2,000 milligrams—oral or parenteral (injected). Subsequent maintenance doses of 100 to 300 milligrams daily are usually sufficient to keep the urine free from these deposits. It would thus appear that deficiency of vitamin C, which is the predominating factor in the various 'stone areas' (of the world) may provide the predominating factor in urinary lithogenesis (stone formation)."

In other experiments done over past years, large doses of vitamin C were not found to increase one's excretion of oxalic acid. **So, even if oxalic acid should be the cause of bladder or kidney stones, large doses of vitamin C apparently do not produce the oxalic acid which would be necessary for this to take place.** Dr. Stone tells of a number of experiments on animals and human beings in which the increase of oxalic acid being excreted was, in fact, much smaller than the differences between individuals in their excretion of vitamin C.

Dr. Stone reminds us that vitamin C kills both harmful bacteria and viruses. Why not, he asks, use it for its beneficial effects on urinary infections which are almost universal in this country, especially among girls and women. By taking frequent doses of vitamin C throughout the day, one can continuously bathe the tissues of the urinary tract in vitamin C at high enough levels to destroy bacteria and/or viruses that are present.

Oxalic acid, incidentally, is a natural element in some foods. It is most abundant in those dark, green, leafy vegetables which are so loaded with minerals and vitamin A that you should make them an important part of your meals: lamb's-quarters (the weed with the fabulous vitamin A content), beet greens, purslane (a common garden weed which is very good to eat), spinach, Swiss chard, sorrel and parsley. Rhubarb is also a source of oxalic acid. The very high oxalic acid content of rhubarb *leaves* is the reason these are not recommended for eating. We eat just the stalks.

Down through the ages, our ancestors have been aware that eating large amounts of oxalate-rich food, to the exclusion of other wholesome foods, may cause trouble. But, except under conditions of famine, there seems to be no reason why anyone would do this. There are also people with an inherited disease who do not handle oxalic acid as the rest of us do, we are told in *Toxicants Occurring Naturally in Foods*, published by the National Academy of Sciences. But, says this volume, "The role of exogenous oxalates (that is, oxalates in food) in the production of renal stones seems doubtful in most cases."

There is considerable evidence from unimpeachable sources that **large doses of vitamin C prevent bladder cancer and prevent the return of cancer in those patients who have already been treated for this.** Physicians at Tulane University regularly prescribe 1½ grams (1,500 milligrams) of vitamin C in three doses, spaced throughout the day, for their patients who, "due to age, cigarette smoking or other factors, may be prone to bladder tumor formation."

The other day we were asked whether or not large doses of vitamin C, taken before a urine test for sugar, can throw off the results of the test.

Our opinion comes from Dr. Irwin Stone, who says: "The urinary spillover from large doses of ascorbate will cause interference in the usual screening tests for sugar in the urine (False Negative Tests for Urinary Glucose in the Presence of Ascorbic Acid. J. S. Mayson et. al., *Amer. J. Clin. Path.*, 58: 297-299, 1972). It can also give false positive tests depending upon the particular screening test employed.

"Two years later, the paper entitled, 'A Simple Method to Prevent Vitamin C Interference with Urinary Glucose Determinations' appeared (R. Brandt et. al., *Clinica Chimica Acta*, 51:103-104, 1974).

"The way the ascorbate-interference was eliminated was to pass the urine through a column of anion exchange resin (Bio-Rad AGI-X4 chloride form 200-400 mesh) 5mm x 10 mm held in a medicine dropper. A single pass was all that was needed to completely remove the ascorbate. Testing the residual urine then gave the true glucose values in the Ames Labstix or the Lilly Tes-Tape or with Benedict's Reagent. I tried to get some companies interested in selling disposable plastic columns for use in eliminating this interference, but no one seemed interested, so I gave up because I had more important things to do.

"If a person is unable to conduct this simple step before testing their urine or finding a lab to do it for them, then they should have a blood glucose determination made. This is more precise than the urinary determination anyway, and ascorbate intake does not interfere within the required precision," Dr. Stone said.

If you take megadoses of vitamin C, you may have inaccurate results on tests for sugar in urine. The chemical formula of vitamin C is much like that of sugar. So the laboratory technician may send back a report that your urine contains sugar when it is only a bit of vitamin C that was excreted. So we suggest that you discontinue taking vitamin C if you plan to have urine tests for sugar done in the following several days, or use the suggestion that Dr. Stone has just given.

We have also heard that certain laboratory tests for blood in the stool can also be thrown off by vitamin C in the stool.

This is a test given to many millions of people to determine the effects of drugs and to test for cancer of the colon and other intestinal disorders which might produce blood in the stool.

At a National Institute of Health clinic, an anemic woman was being given this test when the medical team discovered that vitamin C in her stool interfered with the chemical used in the test, so the results were inaccurate. They asked her to stop using vitamin C for awhile. She did and several days later the tests were accurate. A negative test might not reveal some serious disorder which should be treated. So accuracy is important. There is no suggestion in this story that the vitamin C is harmful. It just throws off the chemical test.

Index

C

Cadmium poisoning, 116, 123
Calcium, 85, 92
Calcium gluconate, 114
California Orthomolecular Medical Society, 91
Cameron, Dr. Ewan, 19, 28, 34, 44
Canadian Food and Drug Directorate, 127
Canadian Nutrition Survey, 127
Cancer, 19, 27ff., 44, 71, 91, 99, 101, 105, 115, 122, 123, 124, 147
Canker sores, 78
Carbon monoxide, 107, 114, 123
Cartier, Jacques, 141
Cathcart, Dr. Robert, III, 73, 91
Cells, 31, 72
Cheraskin, Dr. E., 13
Chicken pox, 78, 89, 90, 116
Cholesterol, 63ff., 86ff., 103, 104, 116
Chretien, Dr. Paul V., 32
Chromates, 123
Chromium, 104
Clark, Dr. Randolph Lee, 95, 105
Cleave, Dr. T. L., 96
Cohen, Dr. Max M., 97
Cold, the common, 24, 30, 31, 47ff., 73, 75, 77, 78, 113
Cold sores, 78
Colic, renal, 90
Colitis, 90
Collagen, 7, 38, 39, 41, 43, 45, 84, 141
Colon polyps, 98, 99ff.
Constipation, 104
Contraceptives (see "The Pill")
Copper, 18
Cornell Medical Index Health Questionnaire, 14
Cortisol, 104
Cortisone, 42, 89
Cousins, Norman, 37ff.
Crib Death, 61, 62
Crib Death, 56ff., 113
Cumley, Dr. Russell W., 95, 105
Cysteine, 16

D

Dalton, Dr. Wilson, 13
Davis, Adelle, 92, 93
Deason, Gary, 25
DeCosse, Dr. Jerome J., 99
Depression, 11
Diabetes, 103, 104, 105, 109, 115
Diarrhea, 74, 76, 77, 91, 94, 121, 142
Diehl, Dr. Harold S., 128
Diet, deficient, 7
Diet, high-fiber, 41
Discs, disorders involving, 25, 80ff.
Diverticulosis, 105
Drug addiction, 52ff., 116
Drugs, 16, 38, 70, 97, 107, 123, 126, 129
Dyes, coal-tar, 123
Dymock, Dr. Iain W., 97

E

Ears, disorders of, 93
Edema (swelling), 52
Encephalitis, 44, 105
Enzymes, 45, 109, 111, 124, 137
Esophagus, 95
Every Second Child, 57, 62
Executive Health, 18, 19, 81, 82
Exercise, need for, 84, 114
Eyes, disorders of the, 89, 93, 116

F

Familial polyposis, 99
Fatigue, 12, 13, 90
Fats, digestion of, 64
Fats, polyunsaturated, 61, 68
Fertility, 10
Fever, 40, 142
Fever blisters, 78, 116
Fiber, importance of, 100
Fieve, Dr. Ronald R., 107
Fits, 60
Flu (see "Influenza")
Fluge, Dr. G., 60
Fluoridation, 130ff.
Fluoride poisoning, 130ff.

Larchmont
Preventive Health Library

The Library will consist of the following books, issued as indicated. For quick reference, we have left off the full title of each book, which is "Improving Your Health with Vitamin A," etc.

1978

1. Vitamin A
2. Niacin (Vitamin B3)
3. Vitamin C
4. Vitamin E
5. Calcium and Phosphorus
6. Zinc

1979

7. Thiamine (B1) and Riboflavin (B2)
8. Pyridoxine (B6)
9. Iodine, Iron and Magnesium
10. Sodium and Potassium
11. Copper, Chromium and Selenium
12. Vitamin B12 and Folic Acid

1980

13. Vitamin D and Vitamin K
14. Pantothenic Acid
15. Biotin, Choline, Inositol and PABA
16. Protein and Amino Acids
17. Natural Foods
18. Other Trace Minerals

*The best books on health and
nutrition are from*

LARCHMONT BOOKS

—"New High-Fiber Approach to Relieving Constipation
Naturally," by Adams and Murray; foreword by Sanford
O. Siegal, D.O., M.D.; 320 pages, $1.95

—"Program Your Heart for Health," by Frank Murray;
foreword by Michael Walczak, M.D., introduction by E.
Cheraskin, M.D., D.M.D.; 368 pages, $2.95.

—"Food for Beauty," by Helena Rubinstein; revised and
updated by Frank Murray, 256 pages, $1.95.

—"Eating in Eden," by Ruth Adams, 224 pages, $1.75.

—"Is Low Blood Sugar Making You a Nutritional
Cripple?" by Ruth Adams and Frank Murray, 176 pages;
introduction by Robert C. Atkins, M.D.; $1.75.

—"Beverages," by Adams and Murray, 288 pages, $1.75.

—"Fighting Depression," by Harvey M. Ross, M.D.; 224
pages, $1.95.

—"Health Foods," by Ruth Adams and Frank Murray,
foreword by S. Marshall Fram, M.D.; 352 pages, $2.25.

—"Minerals: Kill or Cure?" by Ruth Adams and Frank
Murray; foreword by Harvey M. Ross, M.D.; 368 pages,
$1.95.

—"The Compleat Herbal," by Ben Charles Harris, 252
pages, $1.75.

—"**Lose Weight, Feel Great,**" by John Yudkin, M.D.; 224 pages, $1.75.

—"**The Good Seeds, the Rich Grains, the Hardy Nuts for a Healthier, Happier Life,**" by Adams and Murray; foreword by Neil Stamford Painter, M.D.; 304 pages, $1.75.

—"**Megavitamin Therapy,**" by Adams and Murray, foreword by David Hawkins, M.D.; introduction by Abram Hoffer, M.D.; 288 pages, $1.95.

—"**Body, Mind and the B Vitamins,**" by Adams and Murray, foreword by Abram Hoffer, M.D.; 320 pages, $1.95.

—"**The Complete Home Guide to All the Vitamins,**" by Ruth Adams, foreword by E. Cheraskin, M.D.; 432 pages, $2.50.

—"**Almonds to Zoybeans,**" by "Mothey" Parsons, 192 pages, $1.50.

—"**Vitamin C, the Powerhouse Vitamin, Conquers More than Just Colds,**" by Adams and Murray, foreword by Frederick R. Klenner, M.D.; 192 pages, $1.50.

—"**Vitamin E, Wonder Worker of the '70's?**" by Adams and Murray, foreword by Evan V. Shute, M.D.; 192 pages, $1.25.

Before ordering books from Larchmont Books, please check with local health food stores in your area. It will save postage and handling costs. If ordering by mail, please include 50¢ extra for each book for postage and handling; mail to Larchmont Books, 6 E. 43rd St., New York, N.Y. 10017.